CSA Scenarios
for the new MRCGP

CSA Scenarios
for the new MRCGP

Frameworks for clinical consultations

Thomas M. Das

MBBS, MRCGP, DCH, BSc (Hons)
GP in London

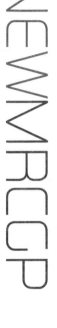

Scion

First published 2009
Reprinted 2009, 2010

A CIP catalogue record for this book is available from the British Library.

ISBN 978 1 904842 64 4

Scion Publishing Limited
Bloxham Mill, Barford Road, Bloxham, Oxfordshire OX15 4FF
www.scionpublishing.com

Important Note from the Publisher
The information contained within this book was obtained by Scion Publishing Limited from sources believed by us to be reliable. However, while every effort has been made to ensure its accuracy, no responsibility for loss or injury whatsoever occasioned to any person acting or refraining from action as a result of information contained herein can be accepted by the authors or publishers.

The reader should remember that medicine is a constantly evolving science and while the authors and publishers have ensured that all dosages, applications and practices are based on current indications, there may be specific practices which differ between communities. You should always follow the guidelines laid down by the manufacturers of specific products and the relevant authorities in the country in which you are practising.

Typeset by Phoenix Photosetting, Chatham, Kent, UK
Reprinted by Thomson Litho, East Kilbride, UK

Contents

Preface ix
Acknowledgements ix
Abbreviations xi

Section 1 – An approach to the CSA

How to pass the CSA – full marks in 10 minutes 3
Basic consultation structure 4
Consultation structure – summary 8
Interpersonal skills 9
What if your mind goes blank? 10

Section 2 – Special GP cases

Breaking bad news 15
The angry patient and complaints 17
Patient refusing emergency management 19
Mental Capacity Act 20
Patients under 16 21
Domestic violence 22
Palliative care 23

Section 3 – Typical cases
Cardiovascular
Cardiovascular lifestyle advice 27
Hypertension 28
Hypercholesterolaemia 30
Chest pain 32
Angina 33
Palpitations 34
Intermittent claudication 36
Varicose veins 37

Respiratory
Smoking cessation 39
Cough 40
COPD 42
Asthma 45

Gastro-intestinal
Obesity 49
Drugs and surgery for obesity 51
Dyspepsia 52
Irritable bowel syndrome 54
Rectal bleeding 56
Constipation 57
Diarrhoea 58
Pruritus ani 59
Anaemia 61

Liver disease 63
Inguinal hernia 64

Endocrinology
Diabetic review 65
Type 2 diabetes mellitus 67
Goitre 69
Tired all the time 71
Thyroid disease 73
Chronic fatigue syndrome 74
Gynaecomastia 76

Musculo-skeletal
Osteoporosis 79
Carpal tunnel syndrome 81
Joint pain – general approach 83
Back pain 85
Knee pain 87
Shoulder pain 89
Polmyalgia rheumatica 90
Neck pain 91
Osteoarthritis 92
Gout 94
Tennis elbow 95
Raynaud's phenomenon 97
Dupuytren's contracture 99

Neurology
Headache 101
Migraine 102
Transient ischaemic attack 104
Head injury 106
Collapse 107
Falls 108
Parkinson's Disease 110
Dementia 112

Dermatology
Fungal skin infections 113
Acne 115
Eczema 116
Psoriasis 118

ENT
Ear pain 121
Tinnitus 122
Dental pain 123
Labyrinthitis / vestibular neuronitis 124
Snoring 126

Ophthalmology
Painful and red eye   127

Genito-urinary and men's health
Prostate-specific antigen   129
Haematuria   130
Erectile dysfunction   132
Benign prostatic haemoplasia   134
Urinary incontinence   136
Testicular pain   138

Renal
Chronic kidney disease   139
Management of CKD in primary care   141

Women's health
Menorrhagia   143
Amenorrhoea / oligomenorrhoea   145
Premenstrual tension   146
Polycystic ovary syndrome   147
Hirsutism   148
Combined oral contraceptive pill   149
Emergency contraception   151
Termination of pregnancy request   153
Subfertility   155
Screening   157
Diagnosing menopause   158
Starting hormone replacement therapy   159
Antenatal counselling   161
Booking visit   163
Subsequent antenatal visits   164

Paediatrics
General approach   165
ADHD   166
Nocturnal enuresis   167

Psychiatry
Depression   169
Anxiety   171
Psychiatric risk assessment   173
Recent non-accidental overdose   174
Alcoholism   176
Insomnia and sleep disorders   178
Eating disorders   180
Opiate addiction   182
Cannabis abuse   184
Post-traumatic stress disorder   185

Appendices
Appendix 1 – Influenza and pneumococcal vaccination, AAA screening   187
Appendix 2 – History taking   189

Preface

This book is based upon the set of notes I compiled and used to pass the Clinical Skills Assessment (CSA) part of the new MRCGP. In the following pages over 100 cases are presented in a structured format optimised for exam success.

I found that the real difficulty was not only gathering vast amounts of information from up-to-date sources into a consultation structure, but also to distil it so the case can be completed in 10 minutes.

Therefore this book aims to:
1. provide up-to-date information in a concise, structured and accessible manner
2. enable the candidate to complete the case in 10 minutes

While this book is not a comprehensive textbook of medicine, I have included summaries of certain "hot topics" where appropriate.

So use the cases, make sure you see plenty of real patients and practise, practise, practise.

Good luck!

Thomas M. Das
August 2008

Acknowledgements

Thank you to Jonathan Behr, Robin Clark, Serena Foo, and Aisha Laskor for your helpful comments and feedback.
Thank you to Mark Sweeney for being an inspirational mentor.
Thank you to my dad for giving me the opportunity to study medicine.
The biggest thanks go to my wife Thao for, amongst other things, putting up with me during all these years of medical training.

Dedication

I dedicate this book to my mum for her bravery and love, and for encouraging me to always follow my heart. Thank you.

Abbreviations

A2RA	Angiotensin 2 receptor antagonists
AAA	Abdominal aortic aneurysm
A&E	Accident and emergency department
ACEi	ACE inhibitor
AF	Atrial fibrillation
BMI	Body mass index
BP	Blood pressure
BPAD	Bipolar affective disorder
CBT	Cognitive behavioural therapy
CCF	Congestive cardiac failure
CHD	Chronic heart disease
CI	Contraindication
COCP	Combined oral contraceptive pill
COPD	Chronic obstructive pulmonary disease
CKD	Chronic kidney disease
CRF	Chronic renal failure
CRP	C-reactive protein
CSA	Clinical skills assessment
CSF	Cerebro-spinal fluid
CVD	Cardiovascular disease
CVS	Cardiovascular system
CXR	Chest X-ray
DH	Drug history
DM	Diabetes mellitus
DSH	Deliberate self harm
DVLA	Driver and Vehicle Licensing Agency
DVT	Deep vein thrombosis
ECG	Electrocardiogram
ESR	Erythrocyte sedimentation rate
FBC	Full blood count
FEV1	Forced expiratory volume in 1 second
FSH	Follicle stimulating hormone
FVC	Forced vital capacity
GCS	Glasgow Coma Scale
GFR	Glomerular filtration rate
GI	Gastro-intestinal
GMC	General Medical Council
GORD	Gastro-oesophageal reflux disease
GTN	Glyceryl trinitrate
GU	Genito-urinary
Hb	Haemoglobin
IBD	Inflammatory bowel disease

IBS	Irritable bowel syndrome
ICE	Ideas, concerns and expectations
IMB	Inter-menstrual bleeding
IVDU	Intravenous drug user
LA	Local anaesthetic
LFTs	Liver function tests
LOC	Loss of consciousness
LRTI	Lower respiratory tract infection
MCS	Microscopy, culture and sensitivities
MSU	Mid-stream urine
NAI	Non-accidental injury
NICE	National Institute for Health and Clinical Excellence
NRT	Nicotine replacement therapy
NSAID	Non-steroidal anti-inflammatory drug
NTDs	Neural tube defects
OA	Osteoarthritis
OTC	Over-the-counter
PCB	Post-coital bleeding
PE	Pulmonary embolism
PEFR	Peak expiratory flow rate
PID	Pelvic inflammatory disease
PND	Paroxysmal nocturnal dyspnoea
PO	*Per orum*
POP	Progesterone only contraceptive pill
PPI	Proton pump inhibitor
PR	*Per rectum* (examination)
PTSD	Post-traumatic stress disorder
PVD	Peripheral vascular disease
RA	Rheumatoid arthritis
RICE	Rest, ice, compression, elevation
RR	Respiratory rate
RVF	Right ventricular failure
SE	Side effect
SOB	Shortness of breath
SSRI	Selective serotonin reuptake inhibitor
STI	Sexually transmitted infection
Sz	Schizophrenia
T2DM	Type 2 diabetes mellitus
TFTs	Thyroid function tests
TIA	Transient ischaemic attack
U&Es	Urea and electrolytes
URTI	Upper respiratory tract infection
USS	Ultrasound scan
VTE	Venous thrombo-embolism

Section 1
An approach to the CSA

How to pass the CSA – full marks in 10 minutes

Each case is marked using three equally weighted domains:
1. data gathering
2. management
3. interpersonal skills

The key is to complete all of the above domains for all cases competently within the allocated 10 minutes. Here are the five key steps needed to do this.

The five key steps
1. Initial open question
2. Targeted history with red flags/examination
3. Ideas, concerns, expectations (ICE) and effect on day-to-day life
4. Explain diagnosis and shared management plan
5. Safety net / arrange follow up

Keeping to this basic structure will ensure all domains are covered. The red flags and safety net ensure the consultation is safe.

All five steps pose a challenge to the CSA candidate, but most find steps 2 and 4 especially difficult. Therefore while this book covers all five steps, it goes into more detail on steps 2 and 4.

During the exam
Writing down the five key steps on the notepaper provided in the exam will prompt you to cover all three domains regardless of your nerves

Interpersonal skills will be demonstrated throughout the 10 minutes.

Each step, together with interpersonal skills will be expanded in the next sections.

It is important to verbalise what you are thinking in the exam. You cannot obtain marks for unspoken thoughts, for example, if you are concerned about patient's safety at home or are unsure if they understand what is being said. Similarly, if you offer to give written information, you will only gain marks if you have explained the contents of written materials.

Basic consultation structure

This section expands on the five key steps outlined in the previous section.

1. Initial open question

"Hello, my name is Dr X... How can I help today?"

Then actively listen: make eye contact, gently smile and nod whilst listening.

The actor will volunteer a set amount of information. In some cases, this will purposefully not be very much. Follow up with a second open question you already have up your sleeve:

"Could you tell me more about ....?"
Very occasionally a third open question will be needed; try:

"How did it all begin?"

Initial open questions
These three simple open questions can be lifesavers during the CSA:
1. *"How can I help today?"*
2. *"Can you tell me more about ....?"*
3. *"How did it all begin?"*

---

2. Targeted history with red flags / examination

Try to cover all the main headings in the table below for each case. Often most of the information will already be covered in the patient summary sheet. However, it is possible that not all relevant information will be given, thus reflecting real life (e.g. smoking status in patient with raised blood pressure).

Targeted history	Key questions
Presenting complaint	*"What do you mean by 'migraine'?"*
History	*"Have you ever had this before?"* *"Have you already tried anything?"* *"Why present now?"*
Past medical history, family history, and drug history	Drug concordance, OTC/herbal remedies

Targeted history	Key questions

Social history
    Home/work/relationships
    Smoking/alcohol/recreational drugs
    Driving
	Who lives at home?
	How are things at work? Outside work?
	Has anything happened at home/work?

Red flags	Weight loss Bleeding (PO/PV/PR/GU) Pain (chest, bone, …)

During the exam – red flags
Red flags are worrying features which are specific to the condition, but a simple rule is to ask about weight loss, bleeding and pain.

Examination for red flags and specific signs only if case requires – see later chapters for more information on this.

3. ICE and effect on life

ICE (ideas, concerns, expectations)
"Do you have any idea what is causing this?"
"Is there anything in particular that you are concerned about?"
"Is there anything in particular you were hoping I could do for you today?"

Effect on life
"How does this affect your day-to-day life?"
   and/or
"Does it stop you from doing anything"

For most cases, it is important to ensure that all these four questions are asked at some point. When to ask which question will vary depending upon the presenting complaint.

For psychiatric and social type cases, it is often useful to ask about ideas early. This can also be used if you are stuck (see also *"What to do if your mind goe'* section below).

4. Explain diagnosis and shared management plan

This step is one of the most difficult parts of the CSA, and is part of what this book is about. The approach will vary depending on the type of case, but there are some suggested guidelines.

Use jargon free language
Try to use the same words as the patient if possible. The specific cases in *Section 3* provide advice on this.

Tell the patient your diagnosis
Check their understanding of this (ideas).

Give management options
Often there will be more than one option, but sometimes it will be necessary to recommend urgent management (if the patient has red flags). Give rationale for investigations and treatments where appropriate, especially if urgent management is needed.

Involve the patient in the 'shared management plan'
Address the patient's ideas, concerns and expectations (ICE) as well as the effect on the patient's day-to-day life.

Ask the patient what they think of the diagnosis and management plan. Check the patient's understanding, e.g. do they already have an idea of what the treatment options are?

If you are breaking bad news, see *Section 2*.

Possible investigations

Bedside	Urine dip and MCS, infection swab, sputum
Blood tests	FBC, U&Es, …
Imaging	CXR, ultrasound, ECG

Management options

Conservative • specific • social • lifestyle	Wait and see Physiotherapy, relaxation exercises, psychology Inform DVLA, sick note Weight loss, smoking cessation, alcohol reduction, healthy diet, exercise
Medical	Analgesia, PPI, antihypertensives
Surgical	Joint injections, minor and major surgery

5. Safety net and arrange follow up

Tell patient when to seek help, e.g. if not improving in 4–6 weeks, if concerned or red flags. Arrange follow up either with yourself or another health care professional (e.g. nurse, specialist). Refer if appropriate.

Consultation structure – summary

The five key steps

1. Initial open question
2. Targeted history with red flags
3. Ideas, concerns, expectations (ICE) and effect on day-to-day life
4. Explain diagnosis and shared management plan
5. Safety net / arrange follow up

Data gathering

Introduction	Open question
History	Presenting complaint Past medical history Family history Drug history
Social history	Home, job, relationships, smoking, alcohol, drugs
Red flags	Bleeding, pain, weight loss
Examination	If required

Interpersonal skills

ICE	Effect on daily life
For patient	Explain diagnosis

Management

Investigations	Urine, bloods, imaging
Management options	Conservative, medical, surgical Lifestyle, social
Safety net	Arrange follow up

Interpersonal skills

Whole books have been written on consultation skills, but in-depth knowledge of the various models is not required to pass the CSA. Here are some straightforward practical pointers to get you through.

General pointers

Non-verbal: eye contact, smile, active listening.

Verbal: speak clearly, soft tone of voice.

Pick up cues

Non-verbal: *"you seem upset..."*

Verbal: *"you mentioned you look after your grandmother..."*

Empathy

- *"That must be very difficult for you..."*
- *"Sounds like you've been through a lot..."*
- *"I'm so sorry to hear that..."*
- *"I understand that must be quite annoying for you..."*

Specific points

- ICE – address patient's ideas, concerns and expectations.
- Social context of symptoms: effect on work, home, relationships.
- *"How are you coping with it all?"*.
- Don't blame another member of staff if the patient is complaining.

What if your mind goes blank?

There are several strategies.

1. Practise by role-playing

This is essential. The more you practise cases with colleagues, the less your mind will go blank – the book *Consultation Skills for the new MRCGP* by Prashini Naidoo will help with this.

2. Open questions

This strategy is more useful at the beginning of the consultation:

"Could you tell me more about this?"

"How did it all begin?"

"Do you have any ideas what could be causing this?"

3. Summarise

This strategy is more useful if you get stuck during history taking. Tell the patient what you know so far. The process of going through this out loud is often enough to jolt your mind back into being the history taking machine that you already are.

4. Use the five key steps

Here's where it can be useful to note the five key steps at the beginning of the CSA when you are arranging your equipment.

5. Go through the history

Ensure you have covered history of the presenting complaint, past medical history, family history, drug history, social history (including work, home, smoking, alcohol, driving).

People often forget family history, driving, and effect on life. How relevant these are will vary from case to case.

For pain, use SOCRATES (**s**ite, **o**nset, **c**haracter, **r**adiation, **a**lleviating factors, **t**ime course, **e**xacerbating factors, **s**everity).

During the exam – what if your mind goes blank?
Write down the following two lists on a blank piece of paper just before the exam. A quick glance at this when you are stuck will get you going again.

List 1: The History
- History of presenting complaint (HPC)
- Past medical history (PMH)
- Drug history (DH)
- Family history (FH)
- Social history (SH)

List 2: The Steps
- Initial open question
- Target history with red flags/examination
- Ideas, concerns, expectations (ICE) and effect on day-to-day life
- Explain diagnosis and shared management plan
- Safety net/arrange follow up

Section 2
Special GP cases

Breaking bad news

Data gathering

Introduction	Ensure quiet surroundings, private setting, etc *"How can I help today?"*
Patient's understanding	*"Before we start, I wanted to ask you...* *...what is your understanding of the tests and why they were done?"*
Symptoms	Clarify patient's symptoms if relevant, e.g. diabetes, thyroid
Warning shot	*"Unfortunately the test results have come back ... "* or *"The test results do show some abnormal findings"* <then pause>
Break news	*....they show you have <hyperthyroidism>"*
General health	PMH, DH, FH
Social history	Family, relationships Support networks *"who's at home?"* Smoking, alcohol Occupation, driving
Examination	For example, BP, weight, urine

Interpersonal skills

ICE	Clearly explain diagnosis, avoid jargon, use patient's own words How much information to give depends on emotional response of patient
'Chunk 'n' check'	Give information to patient in smalls 'chunks' then 'check' their understanding, e.g. *"what will you tell your wife when you go home?"* Don't talk too much, allow patient to gather thoughts and speak Give time for patient to ask questions
Empathy	Acknowledge patient's emotions and feelings *"It must be difficult for you..."* Soft caring tone of voice, eye contact, open body language

Management

Investigations	As necessary
Management	Negotiate management plan *with* patient Offer written information Lifestyle advice, e.g. stop smoking Conservative, medical, surgical and social management as necessary
Safety net	Allow telephone access Arrange follow-up and support patient, often multiple consultations required Referral as indicated

The angry patient and complaints

General points	Remain professional and calm Try not to be defensive or aggressive Attempt to diffuse the situation Listen and be attentive, allow patient to speak Do not blame others, e.g. *"The hospital/nurse is so disorganised"*
Ask questions	Be inquisitive – this allows patient to voice their concerns and also stops the doctor from being defensive: • why is patient unhappy? • what exactly happened?
Apologise	Even if you have done nothing wrong you can apologise, e.g. *"I'm sorry you had to go though that"*
Acknowledge and empathise	This makes the patient feel heard and allows them to vent their anger This can be done in several ways: • summarise their concern – *"So you waited 10 weeks for the appointment?"* • acknowledge emotion – *"I can see that made you angry"* • empathise – *"It's very annoying to wait so long"* • thank the patient – *"Thank you for bringing this to my attention"*
What does patient want?	Find out what they want *you* to do, e.g. *"Is there anything in particular you were hoping I could do?"*
Plan	Emphasise your commitment to helping the patient and ensure there are no other issues that have not been dealt with • *"I will raise this at a practice meeting"* • *"Let's see if we can stop this occurring again"*
Formal complaint	Direct patient to official complaints procedure if appropriate – *"Would you like to register a formal complaint?"*

Complaints procedure

- Rapid acknowledgment
- Explanation and apology
- How it will be put right
- In writing on practice leaflet

The abusive patient

- The patient's need to be heard is balanced against the doctor's right not to be abused or insulted
- *"I am trying to listen to you but can't whilst you are using such bad language"*
- *"Maybe it would be better to do this at another time when you are less offensive"*
- This may need repeating

Patient refusing emergency management

Capacity	Does patient have capacity to make *this* decision? E.g. if they are hypoglycaemic or intoxicated they may well not
Give advice	Clearly explain what your advice is, e.g. *"My advice is to call an ambulance"*
Consequences	Clearly explain consequences of not following advice, e.g. *"You may suffer irreversible heart damage and there is a risk of death"*
Clarify patient's understanding	This is part of assessing capacity and must be done for both your advice and consequences – avoid jargon
Repeat	The advice may need to be repeated
Documentation	Ensure event fully documented Obtain patient's signature if appropriate

Tips:
- There is usually no need to adopt a forceful tone of voice, and this often just scares the patient and fuels any denial process.
- Show empathy and demonstrate that your advice is in patient's best interests.

Mental Capacity Act

Came into force in UK in April 2007

This is a two-part test. To lack capacity, patient must:

1. have impairment of mental functioning, and
2. fail (any one of the below) to understand the information relevant to the decision:
   * to retain the information relevant to the decision
   * to use or weigh the information, or
   * to communicate the decision (by any means)

Principles:
* a presumption of capacity
* patient has the freedom to make unwise decisions
* if the patient lacks capacity, the decision made on their behalf must be:
  * in the best interests of patient
  * the least restrictive alternative
  * maximising decision-making capacity

Patients under 16

"The duty of confidentiality owed to a person under 16 is as great as that owed to any other person"

BMA, RCGP

Any competent young person, regardless of age, can independently seek medical advice and give valid consent to medical treatment.

Competency

The patient must be able to understand:
- the options – nature, purpose, risk
- the consequences of each treatment and of non-treatment

Encourage the patient to speak to parents *"...and explore the reasons if the patient is unwilling to do so"* (GMC).

Explain to the patient that:
- a doctor is legally obliged to discuss the value of parental support
- they will respect their confidentiality

A doctor must always act in the best interests of the patient.

Patients have the option of registering with another GP for contraceptive services only.

Confidentiality

Confidentiality must be respected except in the most exceptional circumstances, for example, where the health, safety or welfare of someone other than the patient would otherwise be at serious risk.

Doctor can breach confidentiality if ALL of below are met:
- the patient does not have sufficient understanding (lacks competence)
- the patient cannot be persuaded to involve an appropriate person in the consultation
- it is in the best interests of the patient

So, even if the patient lacks competence, try to maintain confidentiality unless it is not in the patient's best interests.

In exceptional circumstances where a doctor chooses to break confidentiality, the doctor must:
1. try to convince the patient to voluntarily give information first
2. be prepared to justify his or her decision before the GMC

Domestic violence

Based on RCGP guidance

Emphasise confidentiality	
Lead question	*"Do you ever feel afraid of your partner?"*
Ask about domestic violence	*"Have you ever been subject to violence at home?"*
Allow patient to tell story	
Provide information	*"Violence in the home is as illegal as violence in the streets"*
Safety plan	Do not pressurise into any specific action Encourage and respect the patient's autonomy

- Accurate documentation is essential.
- Photographs should be taken of all patients with visible injuries.

Palliative care

Screen for depression and anxiety (and treat!).
Make sure carers / family are ok too.
Remember district nurses, Macmillan nurses, hospice, social services, benefits.

Quality and Outcomes Framework (UK)

Discuss palliative care patients 3-monthly at practice meetings.

Pain

Mild: paracetamol, ibuprofen.
Moderate: Diclofenac 50 mg tds, co-codamol 30/500.
Severe: Oramorph = morphine sulphate elixir 10 mg / 5 ml
- give with laxative, treat any nausea
- start at 5 mg (2.5 ml) 4-hourly, aim for complete analgesia (no breakthrough pain)
- titrate by increasing dose (not interval)
- once pain control achieved, divide 24 h dose by 2 and give as MST 12-hourly
- as tolerance occurs, add Oramorph (elixir), then total 24 h dose again once control achieved
- use suppositories, patches or injections if unable to swallow

Gastric distention: try antacid or domperidone 10 mg tds.
Bowel colic: loperamide or hyoscine hydrobromide.
Muscle spasm: baclofen, diazepam.
Bone pain: opiates are usually required, NSAIDs, radiotherapy.
Nerve compression pain: dexamethasone if due to inflamation, radiotherapy.
Neuropathic pain: tricyclic acid, gabapentin, pregabalin.

Controlled drugs

Know where to look in *BNF*.

Anorexia

Causes: depression, drugs, nausea, obstruction, sore mouth.
Treatment: small feeds, small plate, prednisolone 15–30 mg daily.

Vomiting

Causes: obstruction, drugs (chemotherapy, opiates), raised ICP, renal failure, hypercalcaemia.
History and examination: headache, micturition, papilloedema, obstruction.

Investigations: U&Es, Ca.
Management: prochlorperazine (buccal, PO, PR, im), metoclopramide, cyclizine, domperidone.

Hiccups

Treat any gastric distention with antacid, metoclopramide, baclofen.

Anxiety

Manage cause, involve carers / district nurse / Macmillan nurses.
Citalopram 20 mg od, diazepam 2–5 mg tds, temazepam for insomnia.

Constipation

Causes: opiates, obstruction, immobility, dehydration.
Beware the patient in overflow, e.g. on morphine with diarrhoea.
Management: lactulose, movicol, senna, gycerol suppositories, phosphate enema.

Cough

Management: steam inhalation, codeine linctus, Oramorph.

Depression

Low index of suspicion, involve carer / district nurse, ensure carers / family well supported.

Dyspnoea

Exclude pneumonia, effusion, bronchospasm.
Consider prescribing morphine, diazepam.
Secretions: hyoscine, atropine.
Bronchospasm: dexamethasone.

Section 3
Typical cases

Cardiovascular lifestyle advice

Adapted from NICE guidelines

Diet	Fat <30%, high polyunsaturated fats, low saturated fats Five portions fruits and vegetables Do not routinely recommend omega 3, or plant sterols
Exercise	30 minutes moderate intensity physical activity a day, at least 5 days a week, or at safe maximum capacity (if co-morbidities), e.g. cycling, brisk walking, stairs Shorter bouts of physical activity of 10 minutes or more accumulated throughout the day are as effective as longer sessions of activity Agree goals, provide written information
Weight loss	
Smoking cessation	
Alcohol	<14 units women, <21 units men per week, avoid binge drinking
Avoid salt and caffeine	(NICE hypertension guidelines)

Post-MI

- Sexual intercourse when comfortable to do so, usually after 4 weeks; no increase in MI compared to rest of population.
- Encourage cardiac rehabilitation program (stable patients only).

Aspirin

- Recommended at 75 mg/day to all aged over 50 years with 10 year CVD risk >20% and controlled blood pressure (British Hypertension Society) if no contraindications.

Hypertension

Data gathering

History	Usually asymptomatic
	Risk factors
	CVD, DM, smoking, raised cholesterol, family history
Social history	Smoking, alcohol
	Lifestyle – occupation, stress, diet, exercise
Red flags	Diastolic BP >120, microscopic haematuria, encephalopathy, pregnant
	Impending complications, e.g. TIA, left ventricular failure
Examination	Weight
	BP – confirm hypertension with 2–4 readings over 4–6 weeks
	Fundi
	Heart
	Peripheral pulses including aortic aneurysm

Interpersonal skills

ICE	Stress
For patient	*"One of several risk factors that can increase the chance of having a heart attack or stroke"*

Management

Investigations	Urine dip – protein
	Bloods – FBC, U&Es, cholesterol, glucose, urate
	ECG
	Urinary catecholamines if young (phaemochromocytoma)
Management	*Conservative*
	Lifestyle advice, relaxation techniques
	Medical
	Age < 55 years or non-black: ACE inhibitor is first line
	Age >55 years or black: calcium channel blockers or thiazide diuretic is first line
	Other drugs: A2RA, beta blockers, alpha blockers, other diuretics
	Primary prevention – aspirin, statin

Safety net	Confirm high blood pressure with 2–4 readings over 4–6 weeks
	Regular review depending on control and calculate CVD risk
	Refer urgently if suspected malignant hypertension or pregnant
	Refer routinely if young or multiple risk factors

NICE guidelines (2006)

Treat hypertension if sustained BP readings greater than:
- 160/100
- 140/90 if cardiovascular disease, target organ damage, diabetes or 10 year CVD risk >20%

Treatment target BP – aim for BP readings:
- <140/85 (Quality and Outcomes Framework audit standard is <150/90)
- <130/80 if diabetic or cardiovascular disease

Hypercholesterolaemia

Incorporating NICE guidelines (2008)

Data gathering

History	Data gathering is essentially about quantifying cardiovascular risk
	
	Past medical history
	    Hypertension, CKD, DM, CVD, PVD
	Family history
	    CVD with age of onset, raised cholesterol
	Drug history
	    Antipsychotics, HIV treatment
	Non-modifiable risk factors
	    Male, increasing age, South Asian origin

Social history	Smoking, alcohol Exercise
Red flags	Chest pain
Examination	Obesity: BMI (or waist circumference or waist:hip ratio) BP Tendon xanthomas, xanthalesma

Interpersonal skills

ICE	Important to explore ICE so you can build a shared management plan How willing is patient to undergo lifestyle modification or take medication?
For patient	*"A fatty substance made by liver from the fat eaten in our diet. Everybody needs a small amount of cholesterol. Too much can build up in arteries and cause them to narrow. One of several risk factors that can increase chance of having heart attack or stroke"*

Management

Investigations	Fasting bloods: lipids, glucose, U&Es, LFTs, TFTs CK only if muscle symptoms

Management	Calculate 10 year CVD risk if primary prevention

	Conservative
	   Diet, exercise, smoking cessation (see *Cardiovascular lifestyle advice*)
	Medical
	   Statins: simvastatin 40 mg (NICE: currently first line)
	   Ezetimibe
	   Fibrates
	
	   Also: aspirin
	   Treat co-morbidities, e.g. hypertension, diabetes

Safety net	Measure LFTs at 3 and 12 months after starting statin Regular review

Diet

Avoid:
- full fat dairy: butter, lard, ghee, cream, full fat cheeses
- fatty meats, e.g. meat pies, sausages

Less frying and roasting: try steaming, grilling, boiling instead.

Medical treatment

With statins if primary prevention, i.e.:
- 10 year CVD risk >20%
- diabetic, CKD, familial

If secondary prevention, i.e. established cardiovascular disease (MI, angina, TIA, stroke, PVD):
- lower threshold for initiating statin if (NICE guidelines):
  - age >75 years
  - South Asian
  - first degree relative with premature CHD
  - rheumatoid arthritis, SLE, CKD, HIV treatment, antipsychotics
- aim for total cholesterol <4.0 and LDL cholesterol < 2.0 (NICE)
- consider increasing to simvastatin 80 mg if not achieved with simvastatin 40 mg (NICE)

Chest pain

Data gathering

History	Pain history, rest pain, trauma
	Symptoms
	SOB, pallor, cough, rash, vomiting, abdominal pain
	Leg/calf pain, haemoptysis
	Risk factors
	Smoking, COCP, recent surgery/flight/immobility, past
	medical history / family history
Social history	Smoking, alcohol, recreational drugs
Red flags	MI, PE, aneurysm
Examination	BP, pulse, temperature, respiratory distress
	Heart, lungs, abdomen
	Chest wall tenderness
	Legs: DVT, oedema

Interpersonal skills

ICE	Effect on life

Management

Investigations	Bloods: FBC, U&Es, LFTs, ESR/CRP, glucose
	ECG
	CXR
Management	Treat as per cause
	Don't forget gastro-intestinal causes such as GORD
Safety net	Refer urgently to A&E (by ambulance) if red flags

Angina

Data gathering

History	Relief with GTN
	Frequency, previous episodes
	Past medical history
	Hypertension, hypercholesterolaemia, DM
	Family history
	Cardiovascular disorders, smoking
Social history	Smoking, alcohol
Red flags	Rest pain, increasing frequency attacks, suspected MI
Examination	BP, pulse
	Heart, ankles

Interpersonal skills

ICE	Effect on life, occupation
For patient	*"Pain that comes from the heart due to narrowing of its blood vessels"*

Management

Investigations	Bloods – FBC, U&Es, cholesterol, glucose
	ECG, exercise ECG
	CXR
Management	*Conservative*
	Stop smoking
	Diet, exercise, stress reduction
	Medical
	Nitrates – GTN spray, oral nitrates for symptom relief
	Beta blocker – first line treatment
	Calcium channel blocker
	Cardiovascular prevention: aspirin, statin
Safety net	To seek medical attention if red flags, refer as appropriate
	Refer newly diagnosed for exercise ECG to confirm diagnosis

Palpitations

Data gathering

History	*"What do you mean by palpitations?"*
	When does it happen? How long last for?
	How fast? Regular/irregular? Ask patient to tap out rhythm
	
	Associated symptoms
	    Cardiovascular: chest pain, SOB, sweating, loss of
	        consciousness / feeling faint
	    Anxiety: finger and peri-oral tingling (hyperventilation),
	        clarify anxiety symptoms
	Past medical history / family history
	    Cardiovascular risk factors, anxiety
	Drug history
	    Including withdrawal (e.g. benzodiazepine withdrawal)

Social history	Caffeine, alcohol, smoking (especially cigars), recreational drugs Stress, anxiety Occupation Driving
Red flags	Chest pain/MI, syncope, known cardiovascular disease Family history of sudden death (cardiomyopathy)
Examination	BP, pulse Radio-radial delay, cardiovascular examination Signs of heart failure Signs of thyroid disease

Interpersonal skills

ICE	Explore patient's ideas and concerns, effect on life Anxiety – could be cause or effect
For patient	*"Awareness of your own heart beating"*

Management

Investigation	Bloods: FBC, TFTs, glucose, cholesterol ECG Echo if suspect cardiomyopathy

Management	Treat as per cause
	Avoid triggers
	Treat any anxiety
	Reassure if simple occasional ectopic beats or non-pathological
	Notify DVLA if syncope or cardiac cause
Safety net	Refer as per cause

Intermittent claudication

Data gathering

History	Cramping pain in buttock/thigh/calf on walking, relieved by rest Claudication distance *Past medical history* CVD, DM, raised cholesterol, family history
Social history	Smoking
Red flags	Critical ischaemia: rest pain, pallor, paraesthesiae, gangrene
Examination	BP, pulse, weight Heart Legs: temperature, skin, infections/ulcers, peripheral pulses Ankle brachial pressure index

Interpersonal skills

ICE	Effect on life
For patient	*"Pain due to narrowing in arteries that supply blood to legs"*

Management

Remember: risk to the limb is low, risk to life is high

Investigations	Bloods: FBC, U&Es, cholesterol, glucose ECG Ankle brachial pressure index or doppler studies

Management	*Conservative*
	    Smoking cessation
	    Exercise
	    Diet
	    Foot care – podiatry, regular self-inspection
	Medical
	    Cardiovascular prevention – aspirin, statin
	Surgical
	    If red flags or treatment resistant

Safety net	Refer if red flags or interfering with functioning

Varicose veins

Data gathering

History	Pain, aching, itching
	Cosmetic appearance and effect on life
	
	Risk factors
	    Prolonged standing, obesity, pregnancy
	Past medical history
	    Ulceration or phlebitis, DVT
	Drug history
	    COCP, HRT

Social history	Occupation – may involve prolonged standing Smoking, alcohol
Red flags	DVT, abdominal mass
Examination	BMI Abdomen Varicose veins: long vs. short saphenous distribution, thrombophlebitis Venous insufficiency: ulceration, haemosiderin deposition, dry skin

Interpersonal skills

ICE	Why have you come to see the doctor now? Explore patient's concerns and expectations Possible effect on self esteem
For patient	*"Enlarged or dilated superficial veins"*

Management

Investigations	Ultrasound studies

Management	*Conservative*
	    Reassurance that most do not cause problems
	    Weight loss, walking, avoid prolonged standing, elevate legs when possible
	    Support stockings
	Surgical
	    Surgery if troublesome symptoms, e.g. injection, avulsion, stripping, laser therapy
	    Surgical treatment not given on NHS for purely cosmetic reasons

Safety net	

Smoking cessation

Data gathering

History	*"How much do you smoke?"*
	When does the patient smoke? e.g. work, social
	When did they start smoking? Why?
	
	Past medical history / family history
	    DM, hypertension, hypercholesterolaemia, obesity, cancer
	Drug history
	    Contraindications to treatment: epilepsy, psychiatric
	        history

Social history	Any smokers at home/work/in relationship? Stress at home/work/in relationship? Support groups
Previous attempts	What happened? What tried? Any problems with previous treatment?
Motivation	*"Why do you want to give up?"* *"Why now?"* *"Has anything happened to make you want to give up?"*

Interpersonal skills

ICE	*"Was there anything in particular you were hoping I could do?"* e.g. patient may want alternative therapies or hypnotherapy Supportive and motivational relationship?

Management

Management	*"Do you know what management options are available?"*
	Encourage patient to agree on a stop date
	
	Conservative
	    Self-help, encouragement, support groups
	Medical
	    NRT: patches, gum, inhalers, nasal spray
	    Zyban
	    Champix

Safety net	Regular follow up and support

Cough

Data gathering

History	Sputum and colour, frequency, diurnal variation
	Associated symptoms
	SOB, wheeze, chest pain, fever, nasal congestion
	GI symptoms (GORD)
	Leg oedema or pain (CCF/PE)
	Environment
	Precipitant, exercise tolerance, allergy, pets, dust
	Travel, contacts, stress
	Past medical history / family history
	PE/DVT, GORD, atopy (hayfever, asthma, eczema)
	Drug history
	ACE inhibitor
Social history	Smoking
	Occupation
	Stress – can patient cope at home?
Red flags	Weight loss, haemoptysis, lethargy/confusion, >40 years old
Examination	BP, weight
	PEFR
	Pulse, respiratory rate, clubbing, anaemia/cyanosis
	Sinus tenderness, throat, neck/lymph nodes, chest, heart
	Legs if suspect PE/CCF

Interpersonal skills

ICE	Effect on sleep, exercise, job
	Sensitively inform patient if you suspect this could be cancer; this can be done by exploring patient's concerns and demonstrating empathy

Management

Investigations	*Bloods*: FBC, U&Es, LFTs, ESR/CRP
	Sputum MCS
	ECG: CCF, PE
	Spirometry
	CXR, CT chest

Management	Treat cause
Safety net	Refer urgently if potential cancer (under 2 week rule)

Causes of cough

Chronic cough (>4 weeks)	Acute cough
Asthma (nocturnal often)	URTI
Cancer of the bronchus	LRTI/pneunomia (treat with
Gastro-oesophageal reflux	ciprofloxacin if allergic to
COPD	erythromycin and amoxillin)
TB	PE
Post-nasal drip	CCF
ACE inhibitors	Asthma

COPD

Data gathering

History	Consider COPD if persistent: • cough >1 month • sputum: colour and volume • SOB: ?exertional *Exacerbations* How many, time course, symptoms, severity, hospitalisation *Co-morbidities* Depression screen Generally fit and well? Appetite? Exercise tolerance?
Social history	Smoking Occupational: exposure to dusts/chemicals
Red flags	Non-smoker with family history Weight loss, haemoptysis, focal chest signs
Examination	BMI – weight, height Clubbing, anaemia, right ventricular failure, lungs PEFR Inhaler technique

Interpersonal skills

ICE	*"How does this affect your daily life?"* *"Is there any reason you have come to see me now?"* *"How are you coping at home?"* Non-judgemental if patient smokes
For patient	*"Airflow into lungs is obstructed. This is due to lung damage, usually caused by smoking"*

Management

Investigations	Bloods: FBC, U&Es, ESR, LFTs Refer to spirometry for diagnosis CXR (for anyone with chronic cough to exclude lung cancer / other pathology)

Management	Conservative
	Smoking cessation = _"the most effective treatment"_
	Weight loss, exercise
	Chest physiotherapy
	Medical
	See below
Safety net	Regular review

Management of COPD

Consider COPD in any smoker >35 years with cough, sputum or SOB.

Diagnosis is with spirometry:
- diagnose COPD with FEV1:FVC <70%
- reversibility (>400 ml after 200 µg salbutamol) suggests asthma

Refer to chest physician if:
- <40 years
- non-smoker
- severe SOB
- diagnostic uncertainty

Stepwise management
- Offer pulmonary rehabilitation to all with subjective limited functioning (graded exercise, behaviour).
- Lifestyle: smoking cessation, weight loss, exercise.
- Depression screen.
- Vaccinations: influenza, pneumococcal.

1. Short-acting bronchodilator: salbutamol or ipratropium.
2. Salbutamol + ipratropium.
3. Long-acting bronchodilator: beta 2 (e.g. salmeterol) or anticholinergics (e.g. tiotropium).
4. Add steroid if moderate to severe disease (FEV1 <50% predicted).
5. Theophylline or referral.

Trial of inhaled steroids for 4 weeks:
- if FEV1 <50% predicted and >2 exacerbations/year (and symptoms not controlled with bronchodilators)
- continue only if benefit after 4 weeks

Mucolytics (carbocysteine) if chronic cough/sputum:
- continue only if benefit after 4 weeks
- caution in peptic ulceration – may disrupt stomach lining

Treatment exacerbation:
- increase bronchodilators
- amoxicillin 1 week then co-amoxyclav or ciprofloxacin 2nd line for 1 week if no improvement
- prednisolone 30 mg for 5 days

Admit to hospital if unwell (e.g. confused, cyanosed, very short of breath), no improvement on treatment, unable to cope at home.

Refer for:
- home oxygen 15 h/day (improves survival)
- surgery – bullectomy, lung transplant, lung volume reduction surgery

Asthma

Based on the British Thoracic Society / SIGN guidelines (2008)

Data gathering

History	Nocturnal cough, wheeze, SOB, chest tightness
	Exercise tolerance
	Triggers/ allergens
	
	Past medical history
	    Exacerbations, hospital admissions, ITU admissions
	Family history
	    Atopy: asthma, eczema, hayfever
	Drug history
	    Current medications and how often used
	    Use of spacer
	    Compliance
	    Aspirin, NSAIDs, beta blockers

Social history	Smoking – active and passive Occupation *Allergens*: pets, diet
Red flags	Respiratory distress, silent chest, chest pain, uncontrolled symptoms
Examination	BMI – weight, height PEFR Chest Cushingoid appearance Inhaler / spacer technique

Interpersonal skills

ICE	Effect on life: sleep, work, school, sport
For patient	*"From time to time the airways narrow making it difficult to breathe. This is due to airway inflammation of unknown cause, but medications can prevent this happening"*

Management

Investigations	PEFR diary (15% variability over 2 weeks) *Spirometry*: FEV1:FVC should be <70% in asthma Trial of bronchodilator / steroid (15% improvement in PEFR)

Management	Conservative
	Smoking cessation, weight loss
	Education, e.g. "preventers vs. relievers"
	Compliance
	"If we could make one thing better for your asthma, what would it be?"
	Medical
	Short-acting beta 2 agonists as required
	Inhaled steroids
	Long-acting beta 2 agonists
	Leukotriene receptor antagonist
	Oral steroids
	Short-acting beta 2 agonists immediately prior to exercise if exercise-induced
Safety net	Admit if any respiratory distress
	Regular follow up
	Refer if uncontrolled symptoms or suspicion of occupational asthma

Diagnosis

Based on the British Thoracic Society / SIGN guidelines (2008)

- Diagnosis is clinical – reversible symptoms without alternative explanation.
- No need for investigations if high probability based on clinical assessment.
- For children <5 years of age: difficult to diagnose – try watchful waiting or trial therapy.

Clinical features raising probability of asthma

- Symptoms worse:
  - at night and early morning
  - after exercise, allergen exposure, cold air
  - after aspirin or beta blockers
- History or family history of atopy.

Not typical of asthma

- No response to trial asthma therapy.
- Normal examination / PEFR when symptomatic.
- Symptoms with URTI only, with no interval symptoms (viral-induced wheeze in children).
- Isolated/chronic cough with no wheeze or SOB.

Prevention

- Breastfeeding *may* have protective effect on child, and so should be encouraged due to other beneficial effects.

Little evidence for treatment of asthma with the following

- Nutritional supplements, certain baby formulas or probiotics/microbial exposure.
- Homeopathy, Chinese medicines, acupuncture.
- Air ionisers.

Quality and Outcomes Framework (UK)

- Record smoking status if >14 years.
- Confirm diagnosis if > 8 years.
- Annual review.

Obesity

Patients are at increased risk of hypertension, cardiovascular disease, DM, arthritis, varicose veins.

Data gathering

History	"Why do you want to lose weight?" Previous attempts?
Social history	Smoking, job, exercise, diet
Red flags	Eating disorder BMI >40 – very significant effect on life expectancy Organic causes – e.g. Cushing's, hypothyroidism, PCOS
Examination	BP, BMI, waist (at level of anterior superior iliac spine)

Interpersonal skills

ICE	Depression, low self-esteem, stress Binge eating

Management

Investigations	Urine – glucose Bloods – U&E, LFT, glucose, cholesterol, TSH, LH/FSH

Management	"Energy you use must be more than energy you eat"
	
	 Conservative
	     Support and encouragement
	     Diet / dietician
	     Exercise
	 Medical
	     Drugs
	 Surgical
	     Bariatric surgery

Follow up	Weigh no more than weekly, regular follow up

BMI (weight/height^2, kg/m^2)

>25 = overweight, >30 = obese, >40 = morbidly obese

Support

- "10% weight loss will give significant health improvements" = motivation.
- Take slowly and set realistic long term goals.

Diet

- 5 portions of fruit and vegetables per day.
- Grilled + boiled + baked rather than fried.
- Smaller portions, limit snacks.
- Less alcohol.
- Water instead of sugary drinks.

Exercise

- 30 minutes per day for 5 days/week.
- Walking, cycling, group activities – aerobics.
- 'Exercise prescription' – for local health services.

Drugs and surgery for obesity

Anti-obesity drugs

Use in conjunction with lifestyle measures, set target 5% weight loss over 3 months.

Orlistat (Xenical) – better for those with high fat intake

- *"Lowers fat absorption".*
- TDS with or before meals.
- NICE criteria: BMI >30 or >28 with co-morbidity (Type-2 DM, cholesterolaemia, hypertension).
- Continue >12 weeks only if 5% weight loss.
- Can cause reduced absorption of fat-soluble vitamins (A, D, E, K) and reduced COCP efficacy.

CI: malabsorption, breastfeeding.
SEs: flatulence, diarrhoea.

Sibutramine (Reductil) – better for those who cannot control eating

- *"Suppresses appetite".*
- Licensed for maximum of 1 year.
- NICE criteria: BMI >30 or >27 with co-morbidity.
- Monitor BP and pulse 2 weekly for first 3 months, then monthly.
- Stop if BP >145/90 or >10 mmHg diastolic BP rise or 10 bpm pulse rise at two consecutive visits.
- Continue >12 weeks only if 5% weight loss.

SEs: dry mouth, abdominal pain, hypertension.

Rimonobant (Acomplia)

- *"Suppresses appetite".*
- NICE criteria: BMI >30 or >27 with co-morbidity.

CI: psychiatric illness.
SEs: dry mouth, abdominal pain, depression, anxiety.

Bariatric surgery

- NICE criteria: only if BMI >40 or >35 with co-morbidities and other measures failed.
- Needs long-term commitment and follow-up.
- Only works alongside conservative and medical measures.

Dyspepsia

Data gathering

Pain	Relationship to eating/lying down
	Night symptoms, sleep disturbance
	
	Associated symptoms
	    Vomiting/nausea, bloating, burping, chronic cough, taste
	      in mouth

History	*Past medical history*
	    Previous endoscopy / investigations
	Family history
	    Ulcer, cancer, surgery
	Drug history
	    NSAIDS, SSRIs, steroids, nitrates, Ca antagonists,
	      bisphosphonates
	Social history
	    Lifestyle: alcohol, smoking, appetite, diet, exercise

Red flags	>55 years, weight loss, bleeding (PO / PR / malaena), anaemia symptoms Dysphagia, vomiting, abdominal mass
Examination	Weight/BMI Hands, anaemia, abdomen

Interpersonal skills

ICE	Effect on sleep, work

Management

Investigations	FBC, LFT, CRP, coeliac screen – consider before referral

Management	*Conservative*
	    Stress, diet
	    Smoking, alcohol, caffeine reduction
	    Stop NSAIDS, etc.
	Medical
	    Gaviscon
	    Proton pump inhibitor 1 month
	    Can add H_2 antagonist or domperidone
	    Consider *H. pylori* test and treat

Safety net	Referral if red flags or persistent symptoms

Consider alternative diagnoses – e.g. gallstones

H. pylori

- Can initially test serology or faecal antigen.
- Urea breath test to confirm eradication (can prescribe on FP10).
- Treatment – e.g. lansoprazole 30 mg + amoxicillin 1 g bd + clarythromycin 500 mg bd for 7 days.

GORD

- Worse lying flat, acid taste in mouth.
- Elevate head of bed, avoid late eating, smaller meals, (medical treatment as above).
- Diet – avoid fatty foods, alcohol, coffee, citrus fruits.

Irritable bowel syndrome

Based on NICE guidelines (2008)

Very common – 10–20% prevalence.
Emphasis on positive diagnosis rather than exclusion of disease.

Data gathering

Symptoms	Consider IBS if 6 months of:
	    Abdominal pain
	    Bloating
	    Change in bowel habit
	IBS must have either (positive diagnosis):
	1. relief of pain with defecation
	2. altered stool frequency/form (straining, urgency, incomplete evacuation)
	Also: symptoms worse after eating, PR mucus

Red flags	Weight loss, bleeding, nocturnal symptoms, masses (rectal/abdominal) Change in bowel habit for 6 weeks and over 60 years of age Family history of ovarian or bowel cancer, raised CRP/ESR
Examination	Weight Hands, eyes (anaemia, jaundice), abdomen, PR (masses, blood) +/– pelvic examination (ovarian cancer)

Interpersonal skills

ICE	Precipitant – *"has anything happened recently?"* *Stressors* Work/home/relationship
Depression screen	Low mood, anhedonia, anxiety

Management

Investigations	FBC, coeliac screen (EMA/TTG), ESR/CRP *Do **not** do:* Ultrasound scan, TFTs, H_2 breath test, endoscopy, faecal tests (occult blood, ova/cysts/parasites)

Management	Importance of 'self help' in management of IBS

	Conservative
	  Diet
	  Exercise
	  Relaxation and leisure – encourage patient to make time
	    for this
	Medical
	  Antispasmodic = 1st line
	  TCA = 2nd line
	Alternative
	  Do not encourage acupuncture, reflexology, aloe vera
	Psychological
	  Only if no effect of medical treatment for 12 months
	  Try CBT, hypnotherapy, psychological therapy

Follow up	Written info, follow up, refer, inform red flags

Dietary advice for IBS
Based on NICE guidelines (2008)

Regular meals, take time to eat, don't skip meals.
Fluids: 8 cups non-caffeine fluid a day.
Bloating – encourage oats and linseed, reduce other fibre (bread, bran)
Reduce:
- caffeine to 3 cups/day
- fresh fruit to 3 portions a day
- alcohol, fizzy drinks, artificial sweeteners (if diarrhoea)

Medical treatments for IBS
Based on NICE guidelines (2008)

1st line: antispasmodic
Aim for "soft well-formed stool":
- loperamide for diarrhoea
- laxatives for constipation – avoid lactulose

2nd line: TCA, amytriptiline 5–10 mg nocte (up to 30 mg) – analgesic effect
- Follow up after 4 weeks.
- SSRI only if TCA fails.

Rectal bleeding

Data gathering

History	How much bleeding – relationship to stool
	Malaena, any other bleeding
	
	Associated symptoms
	    Anal itching and/or pain
	    IBD: fever, mucus
	Risk factors for piles
	    Constipation, heavy lifting, chronic cough
	Past medical history / family history
	    Bowel cancer, bleeding disorder
	Drug history
	    Aspirin, warfarin, NSAIDs

Social history	Alcohol, smoking
Red flags	Weight loss, change in bowel habit, persistent vomiting, >40 years of age
Examination	Weight, BP, temperature, pulse Anaemia, jaundice, lymphadenopathy Abdomen, PR

Interpersonal skills

ICE	Vital to explore ideas and concerns
For patient	Endoscopy: *"A small telescope with a camera put up into the back passage to ensure there is nothing suspicious that could cause the bleeding"*

Management

Investigations	Bloods – FBC, U&Es, LFTs, ESR
Management	Stop NSAIDs Refer immediately if substantial blood loss, in shock or malaena Refer urgently for endoscopy if red flags (under 2 week rule) Treat anal symptoms
Safety net	Wait and see if <40 years and no red flags – follow up 4–6 weeks Seek medical attention if red flags or recurrent

Constipation

Data gathering

History	*Diet and exercise*
	    Fruit, vegetables, fibre, oral fluid intake
	Obstruction
	    Pain, vomiting, distension
	    Recent/previous surgery
	Genito-urinary
	    Difficulty passing urine
	Drug history
	    Opiates
	Family history
	    Bowel cancer

Red flags	Change in bowel habit, weight loss, bleeding, vomiting
Examination	Weight Anaemia, abdomen, enlarged bladder, *per rectum*

Interpersonal skills

ICE	Effect on life, overflow incontinence, embarrassment

Management

Management	*Conservative*
	    Fibre – fruit, vegetables, cereals, bread
	    Water
	    Exercise
	Medical
	    Lactulose/movicol, senna, glycerol supplements,
	        microenema, phosphate enema
	Surgical
	    Treat fissure or cause

Safety net	Refer if red flags

Diarrhoea

Data gathering

History	*"What do you mean by diarrhoea?"* Frequency stool, loose or watery stools, steatorrhoea Blood in stool *Associated symptoms* *GI*: nausea/vomiting/haematemesis, abdominal pain, fever *GU*: urinary symptoms, haematuria, discharge *Risk factors* Unwell contacts Suspicious food Recent travel *Past medical history / family history* IBD, thyroid disease
Social history	Occupation, alcohol
Red flags	Dehydration, uncertain diagnosis, toxic patient, acute abdomen
Examination	BP, weight, pulse, temperature, jaundice, dehydration Abdomen

Interpersonal skills

ICE	
For patient	*"Infection of digestive system"*

Management

Investigations	Usually none required *Faeces*: ova, cysts, parasites, MCS *Urine*: dipsick, MCS *Bloods*: FBC, U&E, LFTs, TFTs, coeliac screen, ESR
Management	Treat as per cause: *Gastroenteritis*: oral fluids, avoid loperamide (use for social reasons only) *Dysentery*: oral fluids, antibiotics if severe or proven *IBD / coeliac disease*: refer for specialist assessment
Safety net	Inform patient to seek attention if not resolving; blood in stools or red flags Refer urgently if dehydrated, toxic or acute abdomen

Pruritus ani

Data gathering

History	*Threadworms*
	Worms in stool
	Peri-anal rash
	Piles
	Heavy lifting, chronic cough, strain at stool, constipation, rectal blood, anal lumps
	Fissure
	Pain on bowel opening
	Past medical history / family history
	DM, psoriasis, eczema, atopy
Examination	Anaemia, abdominal mass, rectal mass, skin tags

Interpersonal skills

ICE	Washing powders, etc.
	Effect of life

Causes

Threadworms: especially in children (egg deposition causes itch – treat child or whole family).
Local: haemorrhoids, fissures.
Infection: fungal (beware DM, immunosupression).
Skin: psoriasis, contact dermatitis.

Treatment

Infections
- Wash hands and nails after visiting toilet (prevent worms).
- Dry peri-anal area after bowel opening and keep clean.
- Avoid irritants/allergens (could be treatment cream).
- Try empirical treatments
  - Threadworms (mebendazole 100 mg stat., repeat after 2 weeks if re-infection).
  - Try hydrocortisone +/– antifungal ointment nocte.

Fissure
- *Conservative*: high fibre diet/lactulose to allow fissure to heal.
- *Medical*: steroid/LA suppositories before opening bowels (e.g. Sheriproct); GTN ointment relieves anal muscle spasm pain.
- *Surgical*: anal stretch, partial internal sphincterotomy.

Haemorrhoids
- *Conservative*: avoid constipation and straining at stool, laxative/high fibre diet.
- *Medical*: steroid/LA ointment or suppository.
- *Surgical*: phenol injection cures 50%; refer for haemorrhoidectomy if 3rd degree, painful++, bleeding++, failed with phenol.

Anaemia

Data gathering

History	*Anaemia*
	    Lethargy, SOB, palpitations, chest pain
	Diet
	    Lack of red meat or green leafy vegetables
	Bleeding
	    Menorrhagia, PO/ PR bleeding, malaena, haematuria,
	      haemoptysis, epistaxis
	Gastro-intestinal symptoms
	    Change in bowel habit, indigestion, vomiting/nausea,
	      abdominal pain
	Chronic disease
	    Renal failure, rheumatoid arthritis, IBD, cancer
	Haematology
	    Easy bruising, infections
	Past medical history / family history
	    Anaemia, sickle cell disease, thalassaemia, thyroid disease

Social history	Smoking Alcoholism Pregnancy
Red flags	Weight loss, bleeding, GI symptoms/signs suspicious of cancer
Examination	BP, weight Palor, pale conjunctiva, koilonychia, glossitis Heart, chest, abdomen – abdominal mass, organomegaly

Interpersonal skills

ICE	Effect on life and occupation
For patient	*"Haemoglobin is a chemical in red blood cells which carries oxygen around the body. Anaemia means there is too little haemoglobin in the blood. There are various causes."*

Management

Investigations	FBC and film, vitamin B12, folate, iron studies Haemoglobin electrophoresis LFTs, TFTs, ESR, coeliac screen
Management	Treat cause Diet, iron supplements
Safety net	If no cause found refer for investigation – usually GI tract for endoscopy If Hb <7 or symptomatic refer for blood transfusion Monitor FBC as per cause

Note

- Exclude B12 deficiency before starting folic acid to avoid precipitation peripheral neuropathy.
- B12 deficiency can cause neurological symptoms (unlike folate deficiency).

Classify anaemia by mean cell volume

Microcytic: iron deficiency, haemoglobinopathies (sickle cell disease, thalassaemia).
Normocytic: blood loss, chronic disease, bone marrow failure, haematological disease, hypogonadism.
Macrocytic: vitamin B12 or folate deficiency, alcoholism, hypothyroidism.
Also: hereditary or haemolytic anaemias.

Liver disease

Data gathering

History	Malaise, lethargy, jaundice, bleeding PO/PR
	Viral hepatitis
	Travel, blood transfusions, sexual history, tattoos, body piercings
	Family history
	Wilson's disease, haemochromatosis, jaundice
	Drug history
	Including over-the-counter preparations
Social history	Alcohol
	Recreational drugs (solvents, mushrooms)
Red flags	Encephalopathy
Examination	BMI
	Well or ill
	Mental state
	Jaundice, signs of liver disease
	Abdomen, ascites, organomegaly

Interpersonal skills

ICE	
For patient	"*Three types of liver disease due to alcohol:*
	• *fatty liver: due to a build-up of fat, reversible upon stopping drinking, no symptoms usually*
	• *alcoholic hepatitis: liver inflammation in which some patients have symptoms depending on severity*
	• *cirrhosis: liver tissue replaced by scar tissue, which causes irreversible damage and loss of function*"

Management

Investigations	FBC, U&Es, LFTs, INR/coagulation screen, glucose, ferritin, copper studies
	Hepatitis screen
	Ultrasound scan of liver
Management	Treat as per cause
	Stop alcohol and hepatotoxic agents
Safety net	Refer as per cause
	Urgent referral if acute liver failure or unwell

Inguinal hernia

Data gathering

History	How noticed? Pain? Reducible? *Risk factors* Chronic cough, heavy lifting, obesity, constipation
Social history	Occupation
Red flags	Strangulation/obstruction – pain, vomiting, distension, absolute constipation (unable to pass faeces or flatus)
Examination	BMI Abdomen, both inguinal regions, external genitalia Often easier to palpate hernia when patient standing up Cough impulse, reducibility, auscultation, transillumination

Interpersonal skills

ICE	Effect on life, concerns Check patient's understanding of what a hernia is
For patient	*"Contents of abdomen protrude through weakness in* *abdominal wall"*

Management

Investigations	Ultrasound scan

Management	Avoid precipitant, e.g. straining
	Weight loss
	
	Conservative
	    Watch and wait:
	• especially if not fit for surgery
	• hernia can enlarge with time
	• explain risk strangulation/obstruction
	• can use truss to keep hernia in place
	Surgical
	    Especially if young or gives history of episodic
	      strangulation

Safety net	Warn patient about symptoms of obstruction Needs hospital admission if obstructed

Diabetic review

Data gathering

Symptoms	"How have you been?"
	1. Energy levels
	2. Polydipsia polyuria
	3. Recurrent infections – skin, genito-urinary, respiratory
	Complications
	    Vision
	    Sensory disturbance, weakness
	    Sexual functioning
	    Chest pain, SOB
	Monitoring
	    Home blood sugar measurements
	    Compliance with treatment

Social history	Smoking, alcohol, diet, exercise Depression screen Driving Occupation
Red flags	Diabetic complications, e.g. DKA, HONK, poor compliance
Examination	BMI, BP, waist circumference Visual acuity and retinal screening Peripheral neuropathy – reflexes, sensation Peripheral pulses Foot care – infections, ulceration, footwear

Interpersonal skills

ICE	Systematic exploration of patient's symptoms; ICE early in consultation
For patient	*"Everyone has small amount of sugar in their blood. In diabetes blood sugar (glucose) is too high. This is due to lack of effectiveness of a hormone called insulin which is made by the pancreas"*

Management

Investigations	Urine – microalbuminuria, albumin–creatinine ratio, ketones Bloods – FBC, U&Es, glucose, HbA1c, lipids

Management	*Conservative*
	    Education, support groups
	    Diet, exercise, smoking cessation
	    DVLA, free prescriptions
	Medical
	    Metformin, sulphonylureas, acarbose, insulin
	Primary prevention
	    Aspirin
	    Statin
	    Control BP
	    ACE inhibitor if microalbuminuria or raised urinary albumin–creatinine ratio

Safety net	Refer as appropriate; regular review

Type 2 diabetes mellitus

Based on NICE guidelines (2008)

Patient education is central to management, ideally as part of a group education programme.

HbA1c

- Ideally aim for below 6.5% but tailor to individual.
- Monitor 2–6 monthly.

Diet

- Tailor to patient's needs, weight loss as appropriate.
- Low fat, low glycaemic index.
- Include low fat dairy and oily fish.
- Discourage foods specifically marketed for people with diabetes.

Medications

- Metformin = 1st line; step up slowly to minimise side effects, monitor U&Es, LFTs.
- Sulphonylurea = 2nd line; warn regarding hypoglycaemia.
- Thiazolidinediones (glitazones) – warn regarding oedema, stop if CCF.
- Exanatide – expensive, if uncontrolled with metformin/sulphonylurea, especially if BMI>35.
- Acarbose – only if other oral agents not tolerated.
- Insulin – if HbA1c >7.5% with all other management.

Blood pressure

- Aim for BP <140/80 (or <130/80 if organ damage – CVD, eye, kidney).
- Monitor 6 monthly if BP raised (annually if no treatment required).
- Lifestyle advice: diet, exercise, weight, low salt, etc.
- ACE inhibitor = 1st line.
- Ca channel blocker or diuretic = 2nd line.
- Ca channel blocker = 1st line if patient may become pregnant.
- Consider starting two treatments initially if Afro-Caribbean.

Blood lipids

- Diet and lifestyle.
- Annual review of weight and CVD risk.
- Offer simvastatin 40 mg if >40 years and type 2 DM.

- Fibrate if raised triglycerides not controlled with lifestyle or statin.
- Aim for total cholesterol <4.0 and LDL <2.0.
- Increase simvastatin to 80 mg or another statin or ezetimibe if target not reached.
- Do not routinely use nicotinic acid or omega-3 fish oils.
- Aspirin if >50 years or raised CVD risk and BP <145/80.

Neuropathic pain

- Tricyclics = 1st line.
- Duloxetine, pregabalin, gabapentin = 2nd line.
- Opiates = 3rd line.

Gastroparesis

- Trial of metoclopramine, domperidone, erythromycin.

Goitre

Data gathering

History	How first noticed, time-course
	Recent illness, pregnancy
	Effect on breathing, swallowing
	
	Diet
	    Iodine deficiency (dairy products, iodised table salt, seaweed)
	Hyperthyroidism: weight loss, anxiety, tremor, palpitations, menstrual disturbance
	Hypothyroidism: weight gain, lethargy, hoarse voice, dry skin, constipation, menstrual disturbance
	Family history
	    Thyroid disease, autoimmune conditions including diabetes

Social history	Smoking, diet
Red flags	Thyrotoxic crisis
Examination	Midline swelling, moves with swallowing Retrosternal extension, thyroid bruit (moves with tongue protrusion only = thyroglossal cyst) Neck, eyes, pulse, tremor, skin/hair Proximal myopathy, reflexes Mental state

Interpersonal skills

ICE	Effect on life
For patient	*"Gland at base of neck that makes a hormone called thyroxine. This thyroid hormone keeps the body functioning (metabolism) at the correct rate"*

Management

Investigations	Bloods – TFTs, thyroid auto-antibodies USS thyroid

Management	*Hyperthyroidism*
	    Refer all cases for specialist diagnosis
	    Propranolol +/– carbimazole for rapid symptomatic relief
	      and prevention of AF
	    May need radioactive iodine therapy or surgery
	Hypothyroidism
	    Refer if young or unwell
	    Oral levothyroxine replacement titrated against monthly
	      TFTs
	    Ensure TSH not suppressed to avoid risk of osteoporosis

Safety net	Urgent referral if thyrotoxic crisis (mortality 10%)

Carbimazole

- Warn patient that they need to seek medical attention if signs of agranulocytosis, e.g. sore throat.

Tired all the time

Data gathering

Clarify symptoms	*"What do you mean by tiredness?"* (physical, mental, malaise)
	 "When are you tired? How long has it been going on for?"
	
	 Ideas
	     Ask early on about ideas
	 Sleeping habits
	     When does the patient go to bed? When do they wake up?
	     Daytime napping? Difficulty sleeping? Refreshed when
	         they wake up?
	 Medical causes
	     Recent illness? Weight loss?
	     Other symptoms? e.g. gastro-intestinal symptoms,
	         exercise, SOB
	     Thyroid disease
	 Psychological causes
	     Depression / stress / anxiety
	 Past medical history / family history
	     Autoimmune conditions, malignancies, neurological
	 Drug history
	     Herbal / OTC

Social history	Alcohol, drugs, smoking, caffeine
Red flags	Unexplained weight loss, bleeding, pains
Examination	Anaemia Thyroid disease

Interpersonal skills

ICE	Ask early on about ideas using open questions *Effect on life* Work, home, relationship, social network Driving, heavy machinery, care of children

Management

Investigations	FBC, TFTs, ESR/CRP Consider CXR – TB, lung cancer
Management	Sleep hygiene Exercise Avoid caffeine and alcohol
Safety net	

Sleep hygiene

- Bedroom for sleep and sex only.
- Wake up same time each day.
- Avoid napping during day.
- Increase daytime exercise.
- Reduce caffeine and alcohol.
- Reduce stimulation before sleep.

Thyroid disease

Hypothyroidism
Weight gain
Lethargy
Hoarse voice
Dry skin + hair
Constipation
Menstrual disturbance

Hyperthyroidism
Weight loss
Anxiety
Tremor
Palpitations
Irritability
Lethargy
Menstrual disturbance

Thyroid examination

Neck, eyes, pulse, tremor, proximal myopathy, reflexes, skin/hair, +/– mental state.

Chronic fatigue syndrome

Based on NICE guidelines (2007)

Data gathering

Key features	4 month history of:
	• new onset fatigue
	• reduction in activity level
	• post-exertional malaise
	Also
	    Sleep disturbance, poor concentration/memory,
	        headaches
	    Flu-like symptoms, muscle/joint pains

Red flags	Weight loss, sleep apnoea, focal neuropathy, arthritis, cardio-respiratory symptoms
Social history	Stress, alcohol, drugs Depression, anxiety
Examination	No lymphadenopathy, no joint swelling

Interpersonal skills

ICE	Effect on life

Management

Investigations	Urine dip
	FBC, U&Es, LFT, TFTs, glucose, ESR, CRP
	Coeliac screen, calcium, creatine kinase
	Ferritin (children and adolescents only)
	
	*Do **not** do (NICE guidelines):*
	    Ferritin in adults, B12, folate
	    Serology (HepB, EBV, CMV)

Management	Cautious optimism: *"Most people will improve"*
	"No known cause or understanding of mechanism of illness"
	Conservative
	Diet – balanced
	Relaxation techniques
	Encourage to continue work/education – stopping is
	detrimental
	Medical
	Tricyclics for poor sleep or pain
	Social
	Talk to family/carers
	Benefits, social support, ME support society
Safety net	Refer for specialist assessment, graded exercise therapy, CBT

Specific management

- Nausea: smaller more regular meals, sipping fluids, drugs as last resort.
- Sleep: avoid daytime napping.
- Limit rest periods to 30 minutes at a time.

Do not offer

- Unstructured exercise – can make condition worse.
- Complementary therapies.
- Vitamin supplements.

Gynaecomastia

Data gathering

History	Normally physiological, i.e. in newborn, adolescence, elderly, obesity
	Duration, tenderness
	Sexual function
	Past medical history
	Liver disease, HIV
	Family history
	Breast cancer
	Drug history
	Digoxin, spironolactone, antipsychotics, cimetidine, anti-retrovirals
Social history	Alcohol, heroin, cannabis
Red flags	Testicular mass
	Suspicious of breast cancer: rapidly enlarging, >5 cm, hard or irregular breast tissue
Examination	BMI
	Is this true gynacomastia? Symmetry
	Liver disease, Cushingoid appearance, signs of hyperthyroidism
	Hypogonadism – secondary sexual characteristics: hair pattern, testicle size, laryngeal size, Klinefelter's syndrome
	Testicular mass/tumour

Interpersonal skills

ICE	Self esteem, effect on life
For patient	*"All men normally have small amount of breast tissue. This is enlargement of male breast tissue"*
	Newborn: *"Due to mother's female hormones (oestrogens) still circulating in newborn. Will get better in a few weeks"*

Management

Investigations	May not need any investigations if obvious cause or physiological *Bloods*: • U&Es, LFT, TFTs • LH/FSH, hCG, oestrodiol, testosterone, prolactin • Karyotype *Ultrasound scan*: testes, breast tissue CXR Fine needle aspiration or biopsy

Management	*Conservative*
	   Treat cause, refer as appropriate
	   Reassure if physiological
	   Weight loss if obesity related
	   May require psychological support
	Surgical
	   If longstanding or fibrosis has developed

Safety net	Refer suspected malignancy urgently under 2 week rule

Osteoporosis

Data gathering

Risk factors	Menopause
	BMI < 18
	Chronic disease: IBD, coeliac, type I diabetes, rheumatoid arthritis, chronic renal failure
	
	Family history
	  Menopause, hip fracture
	Drug history
	  Steroids

Social history	Smoking, alcohol Weight-bearing exercise
Red flags	Hyperthyroidism, hyperparathyroidism, osteomalacia, hypogonadism
Examination	BMI Loss of height Fracture: wrist, vertebral, hip

Interpersonal skills

ICE	
For patient	*"Thinning of bones", "no symptoms"*

Management

Investigations	DEXA scan Bloods: normal FBC, ESR, TFTs, Ca, Vit D, ALP, LH/FSH, testosterone

Prevention (% fracture reduction)	Stop smoking (25%)
	Reduce alcohol
	Weight-bearing exercise (50%)
	HRT (50%)
	Consider stopping steroids
Treatment	Calcium and vitamin D for all at risk of falls or in residential care
	Conservative
	Analgesia and rest for vertebral fractures
	Medical
	Bisphosphonates (eg. risedronate, alendronate)
	SERMS (eg. Raloxifene) – reduces vertebral fracture risk in post-menopausal women
	HRT = 2nd line, early menopause
	Refer for:
	• Calcitriol / Calcitonin / Teriparatide (>65 years, high risk)
	• Strontium (>75 years, high risk)
Safety net	Exclude red flags before treating for osteoporosis

DEXA scan

Offer this if:
- fragility fracture <75 years
- long term steroids <65 years (especially if >7.5 mg prednisolone for 3 months)

Bisphosphonate

"*To slow rate of bone loss*".

"*Swallow with plenty of water whilst upright on empty stomach 30 mins before breakfast*".

Daily, weekly and monthly preparations.

Treat if:
- T score <2.5; or if <1.5 and major risk factor
- steroids and fracture
- long term steroid >65 years
- fragility fracture >75 years (DEXA if 65–75 years with fracture to confirm osteoporosis)

Carpal tunnel syndrome

Data gathering

Symptoms	Tingling and pain radial 3.5 fingers Nocturnal, relieved by shaking Weakness
Aetiology	Idiopathic Pregnancy, menopause Repetitive use, trauma *Rheumatology*: rheumatoid arthritis, scleroderma, osteoarthritis *Endocrinology*: acromegaly, hypothyroidism *Infiltrative*: amyloidosis, sarcoidosis, leukaemia
Red flags	Consider diabetic mononeuropathy Thenar muscle wasting = red flag – refer for decompression
Examination	Weight Tinel's and Phalen's tests Thumb abduction Thenar muscle wasting

Interpersonal skills

ICE	
For patient	*"Pressure on nerve as it runs through the wrist"*

Management

Investigations	Bloods: FBC, U&Es, TFTs, ESR, C-reactive protein, glucose

Management	*Conservative*
	   Rest hand, avoid precipitant
	   Wrist splint – some relief in up to 80%
	Medical
	   NSAIDs
	Surgical
	   Steroid injection
	   Carpal tunnel release

Safety net	Refer if wasting thenar muscles or no improvement in symptoms

DeQuervain's tenosynovitis

- Thumb extensor tenderness.
- Associated with unaccustomed activity, e.g. rose pruning.
- Radial styloid tenderness, thickened tendon sheath +/− swelling.
- Finklestein's test: enclose thumb in a fist and flex and abduct wrist.
- *Treatment*: rest 2–4 weeks, steroid injection, surgery.

Joint pain – a general approach

Data gathering

History	Acute vs. chronic
	Tramatic vs. spontaneous
	Local vs. generalised
	
	Pain
	   Diurnal variation
	   Sleep disturbance
	Other symptoms
	   Stiffness
	   Fatigue, fever
	Precipitant
	   Previous injuries
	   Recent illness

Social history	Depression screen Occupation
Red flags	Weight loss, fever, poor range of movement, poor functioning Neurology
Examination	Joint above and below Look, feel, move, special tests Function

Interpersonal skills

ICE	Effect of symptoms on daily living and occupation

Management

Investigations	Bloods: FBC, ESR, urate, rheumatology screen Joint fluid for microscopy X-ray, ultrasound scan, MRI
Management	Rest, analgesia Gentle mobilisation Physiotherapy if not improving
Safety net	Refer if concerned / red flags

Causes

- Trauma, unaccustomed use, overuse injury.
- Viral illness.
- Rheumatoid arthritis, osteoarthritis, connective tissue disorders.
- Gout.
- Polymyalgia rheumatica.
- Cancers.

Back pain

Data gathering

History	Lifting, trauma Radiation to leg Chronic back pain: depression, carer stress, hidden agenda
Social history	Occupation, finances

Red flags	Age <20 or >55 years
	Pain: nocturnal, thoracic
	Cancer: weight loss, check past medical history
	Oral steroids, HIV
	
	Cauda-equina syndrome
	    Bladder/bowel paralysis or incontinence, leg weakness,
	      saddle paraesthesia

Examination	*Look* *Feel*: tenderness, vertebral steps/alignment, sacro-iliac joints *Move*: flexion/extension, lateral flexion, rotation Straight leg raise + sciatic stretch test (reproduces nerve root pain) Weakness, sensation, reflexes • L4/5: dorsiflexion, extensor hallucis, "walk on heels" • L5/S1: peroneal muscles, toe flexors, "walk on toes" Gait

Interpersonal skills

ICE	Effect on life

Management

Investigations	Bloods: ESR, bone profile, PSA (in the elderly)
	X-ray: ankylosing spondilitis (young), vertebral collapse, cancer (elderly)
	MRI
Management	*Conservative*
	Reassurance, gentle mobilisation, posture
	Physiotherapist / chiropractor / osteopath
	Medical
	Analgesia
	Muscle relaxant (diazepam)
	Social
	Sick note, effect on occupation/life
Safety net	Review 2-weekly
	Refer urgently if cauda-equina syndrome
	Refer if no improvement in 6 weeks

Sciatica

- Pain radiates below the knee, worsened by coughing/sneezing/laughing.

Chronic pain

- Depression screen.
- Treatment support groups, physiotherapy, refer to orthopaedics (surgery) or rheumatology (facet joint injection).

Knee pain

Data gathering

History	Traumatic vs. non-traumatic
	Previous injury
	Range of movement
	Fever, recent illness
	Meniscal damage
	Locking / giving way
Social history	Occupation
	Walking / function
Red flags	Fever, polyarthropathy, urethral discharge, eye symptoms
Examination	Weight, fever
	Look: swelling, redness, effusion
	Feel: tenderness, crepitus
	Move: flexion / extension
	Ligaments, menisci
	Joint above and below: hip and ankle
	Gait

Interpersonal skills

ICE	Effect on life
	Sensitive advice regarding choice of activity may be required

Management

Investigations	Bloods: FBC, ESR, LFTs, calcium, TFTs, RhF, autoantibody screen Fluid for microscopy USS – eg. patella tendon tear X-ray MRI

Management	*Acute trauma*
	    Refer if swelling post injury – X-ray, aspiration
	    If can weight bear and no swelling – RICE (rest, ice, compression, elevation)
	Chronic
	    Footwear
	    Physiotherapy
	    Steroid injection
	    Refer arthroscopy if ligament/meniscal damage
	Condromalacia patallae
	    Analgesia, rest, physiotherapy/quadriceps exercise
	Prepatellar bursitis
	    Rest, analgesia +/– aspiration
	    Admit if cellulitis or pus aspirated
	Osgood Schlatter
	    Tender tibial tuberosity, settles over 2–3 months
	Gout, osteoarthritis, rheumatoid arthritis
	    Treat as per cause

Safety net	

Shoulder pain

Data gathering

History	Trauma Neck pain, neurological symptoms in upper limb Right/left handed
Social history	Occupation Effect on life Driving
Red flags	Dislocation, focal neurology Don't forget: cardiac pain, gallbladder disease, neck pain
Examination	Neck: look, feel, move Abduction/adduction, flexion/extension, internal/external rotation Neurological: power, sensation Painful arc (60–120°) = supraspinatus/rotator cuff problem

Interpersonal skills

ICE	Effect on life

Management

Investigations	Shoulder X-ray Ultrasound scan
Management	Analgesia Gentle mobilisation Physiotherapy Joint injection
Safety net	Refer if suspect fracture, dislocation or nerve damage

Tendonitis: associated with repeated use, settles in 2 weeks, steroid injection.

Rotator cuff tear: suspect if recurrent impingement, refer orthopaedics.

Frozen shoulder: global limitation movement, NSAID, physiotherapy, injection, can take 1 year to resolve.

Osteoarthritis: imaging to rule out other pathology.

Chronic pain: ultrasound scan, bloods (urate, ESR...), refer orthopaedics.

Polymyalgia rheumatica

Data gathering

History	Shoulder pain and stiffness Symmetrical, worse in mornings Hip pain
Social history	Brushing teeth, combing hair, eating and drinking Occupation
Red flags	Temporal arteritis: visual loss, temporal headache/tenderness
Examination	1 in 3 have temporal arteritis Decreased range of movement shoulders +/– hips Muscular tenderness

Interpersonal skills

ICE	Effect on life
For patient	*"Pain and soreness caused by inflammation of large muscles"*

Management

Investigations	Bloods: ESR, TFTs
Management	Prednisolone orally Osteoporosis prophylaxis as appropriate
Safety net	Urgent ophthalmology referral if suspected temporal arteritis

Neck pain

Data gathering

History	Acute vs. chronic Trauma Headache, fever, rash
Social history	Occupation, stress
Red flags	Neurological symptoms: legs and arms
Examination	Neck, shoulder Arms and legs if neurological symptoms

Interpersonal skills

ICE	Effect on life, sleep and occupation

Management

Investigations	C-spine X-ray

Management	*Conservative*
	    Gentle mobilisation
	    Wait and see, physiotherapy
	Medical
	    Analgesia, diazepam

Safety net	Refer if neurological features

Osteoarthritis

Based on NICE guidelines (2008)

Data gathering

History	Pain – diurnal variation Stiffness, precipitant, locking/giving way Current treatment Effect on sleep Depression screen Falls assessment
Social history	Occupation, family life
Red flags	Septic arthritis, rheumatoid arthritis
Examination	Deformity, skin (psoriasis) Range of movement, crepitus Function, gait

Interpersonal skills

ICE	Effect on life, coping at home, carer

Management

Investigations	Bloods: normal FBC, ESR, urate, rheumatology screen X-ray

Management	Three core treatments:
	• weight loss
	• exercise – aerobic and muscle strengthening
	• footwear
	
	Conservative
	    Heat/cold pads
	    TENS
	    Physiotherapy / occupational therapy / walking and other
	      aids
	    Benefits
	Medical
	    Paracetamol and topical NSAID = 1st line
	    NSAID/COX2 inhibitor – prescribe with proton pump
	      inhibitor
	    Topical capsaicin
	Surgical
	    Steroid injections
	    Early referral for symptoms affecting life – joint replacement
	    Knee arthroscopy only for locking

Safety net	

Gout

Data gathering

History	Pain Precipitant, e.g. red meat, alcohol *Drug history* 　Thiazide diuretics, aspirin
Social history	Alcohol, diet
Red flags	Fever, polyarthropathy, alternative diagnosis
Examination	Gouty tophi – ears, tendons Red and inflamed joint

Interpersonal skills

ICE	Effect on life
For patient	*"Type of arthritis caused by build up of substance in blood called uric acid"*

Management

Investigations	Bloods: uric acid, U&Es, lipids Joint aspiration
Management	*Conservative* 　Reduce alcohol, weight loss 　Diet (avoid red meat, fizzy drinks, pulses, oily fish), oral 　　fluids *Medical* 　Stop thiazide / aspirin 　Acute attack: NSAID (e.g. Indometacin) or colchicine 　Prophylaxis: allopurinol
Safety net	Refer to rheumatology if no improvement

Tennis elbow

Data gathering

History	= Lateral epicondylitis Usually unilateral Trauma, repetitive movements, unaccustomed activity Effect on life, e.g. difficulty opening jar
Social history	Occupation, support at home Driving
Red flags	Septic arthritis, neurological symptoms/signs

Examination	Both arms: exclude deformity/swelling/temperature
	Active and passive movements: extention / flexion, supination/
	   pronation
	Sensation and power
	
	Tennis elbow
	   Tenderness at lateral epicondyle
	   Pain maximal on resisted wrist extension

Interpersonal skills

ICE	Effect on daily life
	Diagnosis is usually straightforward, so targeted history and
	   examination are required to have time to explain diagnosis
	   and involve patient in management plan

For patient	*"Soft tissue inflammation of tendons on outside of elbow"*

Management

Investigations	None required
Management	Reassurance and explanation that this is self-limiting and resolves without treatment in most cases Recovery can take several weeks to months *Conservative* Rest, ice, avoid trigger movements Physiotherapy *Medical* NSAID *Surgical* Steroid/local anaesthetic injection Surgical release *Social* Advice regarding safe driving Manage possible effect on occupation
Safety net	Consider alternative diagnosis if atypical history EMG or referral as appropriate if neurological features

Golfer's elbow (medial epicondylitis)

- Similar self-limiting condition with management as above.
- Occasionally associated with ulnar neuropathy.

Raynaud's phenomenon

Data gathering

History	Characteristic history of fingers/toes changing colour: White, Blue, then Crimson (red) (remember: WBC) Triggers: cold, emotion Age at onset *Past medical history / family history* Connective tissue disease (SLE, Scleroderma), Raynaud's *Drug history* Beta blockers, COCP
Social history	Occupation history: work with vibrating tools or in cold weather Smoking
Red flags	Neurological symptoms, connective tissue disease Underlying malignancy – rare
Examination	BP in both arms Upper limb pulses Digital ulceration

Interpersonal skills

ICE	Concerns, effect on life
For patient	*"Due to narrowing of blood vessels in response to a trigger, usually cold weather"*

Management

Investigations	Bloods: FBC, U&Es, LFT, TFTs, ESR, rheumatological screen (RhF, autoantibodies)
Management	Treat underlying cause if found (most cases are idiopathic) *Conservative* Conservative measures usually suffice Avoid precipitant: keep warm, gloves, consider change of occupation Smoking cessation, exercise *Medical* Fish oil, evening primrose oil Nifedipine, alpha blockers, ACE inhibitors *Surgical* Sympathectomy – last resort for severe symptoms
Safety net	Refer if underlying condition found

Features suggestive of underlying cause: unilateral, onset > 30 years, male, digital ulceration.

Dupuytren's contracture

Data gathering

History	Unilateral vs. bilateral, hands vs. feet
	Age at onset, how quickly progressed
	Normally painless
	History of trauma and manual labour
	Past medical history / family history
	Diabetes, high cholesterol, hypothyroidism, HIV
	Dupuytren's contracture
	Drug history
	Anticonvulsant medication
Social history	Smoking, alcohol
	Occupation
Red flags	Sarcoma in young patient – very rare
Examination	Little and ring fingers most often affected
	Thickening of palmar fascia
	Table-top test – can patient place hand flat on to a flat surface?
	Measure contracture at metacarpo-phalangeal joints (MCPJ)

Interpersonal skills

ICE	Effect on daily life?
	Is patient right or left handed?
	Patient's expectations from consultation?
	Opportunity to discuss shared management plan
For patient	*"Fingers bend slowly into the palm of hand"*
	"Due to thickening of connective tissue in palm of hand"
	"Not a dangerous condition"

Management

Investigations	Bloods: LFTs, TFTs, cholesterol, glucose
Management	Consider treating any cause

	Conservative
	    Often no treatment required if mild
	Surgical
	    Usually once flexion greater than 30 degrees at MCPJ or affecting life
	    One hand operated on at a time
	    Warn about possible recurrence

	Most non-surgical methods have very poor results
Safety net	

Note:
- link with Peyronie's disease (penile fibromatosis)
- often idiopathic
- patient usually over 50 years at presentation

Headache

Data gathering

History	Pain score
	Eye strain – spectacles, vision
	Meningism – fever, neck stiffness, rash
	Raised ICP – worse in morning/coughing/sneezing, vomiting, drowsiness
	URTI – associated URTI
	Tension – stress
	Drug history
	Codeine, Ca channel blockers
Social history	Stress at work, home, finances...
Red flags	Sudden onset, severe pain, worsening, >50 years at onset
	Focal neurology, meningism, reduced GCS, head injury, tender temporal arteries
Examination	BP, fundi
	Temporal arteries
	Neck for muscles and movements
	Neuro.

Interpersonal skills

ICE	Depression, stress

Management

Investigations	
Management	Headache diary
	Treat cause
Safety net	Refer if serious features
	Offer follow up

Tension headache: reassurance, relaxation, paracetamol/NSAID.
Cluster headache: 100% oxygen, sumatriptan, prophylaxis (unlicensed: verapamil, lithium).

Other causes of headache

- Analgesia-related.
- Depression.
- Meningitis.
- Tumour.
- GCA/TA/PMR.

Migraine

Data gathering

History	Headache – pain history, unilateral Associated symptoms: • nausea, vomiting, photophobia, phonophobia, wanting to sleep • aura/eye symptoms • focal neurology: weakness/sensory disturbance, dysphasia Triggers factors, e.g. caffeine, chocolate, red wine, cheese, alcohol, stress, fatigue Variation with menses (treat with mefanamic acid) *Drug history* COCP, analgesia
Social history	Smoking, alcohol, stress, sleep Occupation
Red flags	Patient taking COCP and migraine with focal aura or worsening migraines *See also* **Headache**
Examination	Should have no focal neurology between attacks

Interpersonal skills

ICE	Effect on life, concerns Consider depression screen

Management

Investigations	Usually none required
Management	Avoid triggers, relaxation, reassurance Symptom diary *Analgesia +/- antiemetic* 　Paracetamol, NSAID 　Stemetil, Domperidone (Migralieve contains antiemetic) 　Diclofenac and domperidone suppositories available *Triptans* 　Take during headache (not aura) 　Can be oral, subcutaneous injection, or nasal spray 　Contraindications: uncontrolled hypertension, CHD, CVD, 　　<12 years of age *Prophylaxis* 　Propranolol 　Amytriptilline 10–150 mg nocte 　Valproate = 2nd line, unlicensed 　Pizotifen = 3rd line
Safety net	Refer if uncontrolled or uncertain diagnosis Consider stopping COCP Offer follow up

Transient ischaemic attack

Data gathering

History	Vision, speech, weakness, tingling, balance
	Witness, time to resolve (within 24 h), warning symptoms
	Previous episodes
	Associated symptoms
	Headache, chest pain, shortness of breath, palpitations
	Risk factors
	Hypertension, raised cholesterol, DM, smoking, family
	history / past medical history
Social history	Job, driving, smoking
Red flags	Residual focal neurology
	>1 episode in last week
Examination	BP, weight
	Atrial fibrillation, anaemia, carotid bruit, heart murmurs,
	chest
	Neurological examination with cranial nerves
	Peripheral pulses, fundoscopy

Interpersonal skills

ICE	Support at home
For patient	*"Temporary interruption of blood flow to the brain"*

Management

Investigations	Bloods: FBC, BMI, cholesterol, TFTs, LFTs, U&Es ECG Echo, carotid doppler, CT/MRI of brain

Management	*Conservative*
	    Smoking cessation, alcohol reduction
	    Diet: low salt, low fat, fruit/vegetables
	Medical
	    Aspirin 300 mg
	    Dypiridamole for 2 years
	    Statins
	    Control hypertension: ACE inhibitor + diuretic
	Social
	    Inform DVLA

Safety net	Admit if >1 episode in 1 week or focal neurology persists Otherwise refer to TIA clinic within 1 week To seek medical attention if similar symptoms, patient information leaflet Regular follow up

TIA / cerebral vascular accident – regular follow up

- Support, social services, benefits.
- DVLA.
- Depression screen.
- Speech and language therapy, occupational therapy, physiotherapy, social services.
- Annual influenza vaccination.
- Control risk factors: e.g. BP, cholesterol.

Head injury

Data gathering

History	Mechanism and nature of injury, e.g. was patient wearing a helmet?
	Headache, other injuries, bleeding
	
	Past medical history
	    Coagulopathy
	Drug history
	    Aspirin, warfarin

Social history	Alcohol, drugs
Red flags	LOC, amnesia before event, vomiting, drowsiness, focal neurology High impact, >65 years, alcoholism Consider non-accidental injury especially in child <1 year
Examination	Glasgow coma scale, pupils, neurological examination, local injuries Bruising around eyes/ears CSF/blood from ears and nose

Interpersonal skills

ICE	

Management

Investigations	CT head if any red flags
Management	Analgesia: paracetamol, ibuprofen (avoid opiates as you may need to assess pupil size)
Safety net	Refer to A&E if any red flags Warn regarding concussion, give written information: dizziness, headaches, poor concentration, visual disturbance

Consider delayed presentation of *subdural haemorrhage* if: elderly, signs of alcoholism, confusion, falls, memory and balance problems.

Collapse

Data gathering

History	Witness account
	Pre-collapse
	Warning – palpitations, chest pain, sweating, faint feeling, aura
	Precipitant – cough, micturition, standing, exercise
	During collapse
	LOC, duration
	Movements, colour, tongue biting, incontinence
	Injury
	Post-collapse
	Recovery
	Past medical history / family history
	Epilepsy, DM, CVD
	Sudden death
	Drug history
	Antihypertensives, tricyclics, drugs that prologue QT interval
Social history	Occupation Alcohol, recreational drugs, smoking Driving
Red flags	Focal neurology, first seizure, TIA
Examination	BP: lying and standing Pulse, anaemia, heart Neurological examination

Interpersonal skills

ICE	Witness account

Management

Investigations	Bloods: FBC, U&Es, glucose, TFTs ECG
Management	As per cause DVLA
Safety net	Refer first seizure urgently under 2 week rule

Falls

Based on NICE guidelines (2004)

Data gathering

History	Falls: frequency, any witnesses, injuries Vision, continence, dementia Osteoporosis
Social history	Environment / home hazards Daily functioning Alcohol, recreational drugs
Red flags	Exclude organic cause for fall: • memory of fall • warning • associated symptoms • UTI / infection
Examination	Confusion BP, pulse, cardiovascular system Neurological examination: Parkinson's Disease, vision Observe for gait/balance problems "Get up and go" test: rise from chair without using arms

Interpersonal skills

ICE	Address biological, psychological and social issues Fears of falling, fear of being in nursing home Depression Respect patient confidentiality/autonomy if family are involved

Management

Investigations	Urine MCS Bloods FBC, U&Es, glucose, TFTs ECG DEXA bone density scan

Management	Physiotherapy, occupational therapy
	Walking aids: e.g. walking stick/frame
	
	Multi-disciplinary team input
	   Falls centre
	   Strength and balance training
	   Occupational therapy: home hazards
	   Vision test
	   Medication review
	
	Give written information

Safety net	Regular follow up and re-assess risk

Screen all elderly for falls risk.
No evidence brisk walking prevents falls.

Parkinson's Disease

Data gathering

History	Tremor, stiffness, slow movements Falls Can patient cope at home *Drug history* Phenothiazines
Social history	Smoking, alcohol, recreational drugs Social support, family, occupation Driving
Red flags	Depression, anxiety, dementia, not eating Aspiration, infections, incontinence Focal neurology
Examination	Three main features: 1. tremor – resting, pill rolling, 4–6 cycles/second 2. rigidity – cogwheel 3. bradykinesia Shuffling gait with reduced arm swing Expressionless face, drooling Small handwriting (micrographia) Glabellar tap: Parkinson's patients continue to blink Normal power, reflexes, sensation (and coordination in early stages)

Interpersonal skills

ICE	Effect on activities of daily living, carer, 3rd party account Emphasis on holistic care
For patient	*"Disorder of part of brain which helps coordinate the body's movements"*

Management

Investigations	Usually none needed in primary care for diagnosis Bloods: TFTs

Management	Aim is for symptom control, not cure
	
	Conservative
	    Refer early for multi-disciplinary team and neurological
	        assessment and treatment
	    Physiotherapy, occupational therapy, speech and language
	        therapy, social services
	    Driving safety
	Medical
	    Levo-dopa
	    Dopamine agonists: ropinirole, cabergoline
	    MAO inhibitors: selegiline
	Surgical
	    Pallidotomy, thalamic surgery, deep brain stimulation

Safety net	Regular review Ensure patient well supported, support groups Manage red flags, refer urgently if focal neurology, or consider alternate diagnosis

Dementia

Data gathering

Symptoms	Memory, speech
	Personality and behaviour: e.g. aggression, sexual disinhibition
	History from relative / neighbour
	
	Differential diagnoses
	    Deafness, Parkinson's Disease, alcohol, depression
	Past medical history
	    Cardiovascular disease risk

Social history	Support at home Driving Activities of daily living Smoking, alcohol, drugs
Red flags	Focal neurology, trauma, confusion/delirium, abuse
Examination	Abbreviated mental test score: age, time, year, address, person, place, date of birth, WW2, Prime Minister, 20–1 Exclude depression Neurological examination: should be normal Capacity

Interpersonal skills

ICE	Ability to cope at home, continence, sleep Carer and their welfare

Management

Investigations	Urine dip and MCS Bloods: FBC, U&Es, ESR, LFTs, glucose, TFTs, syphilis, B12 In-depth mental state assessment
Management – shared	Referral: for diagnosis / CT head / treatment – preferably with relative/friend Support, social services, nursing home, district nurse, CAB Alzheimer's Society DVLA Independent Mental Capacity Advocate (IMCA)
Safety net	Regular review and reassessment

Fungal skin infections

History	Feet, body, nail, scalp, hair
	Past medical history
	DM, immunocompromise, HIV
	Drug history
	Steroid, antibiotics
Examination	If on fingernails, examine toenails
	Whole skin ideally
Investigations	MCS: skin scraping, nail clippings, plucked hair
	Send especially if considering systemic treatment
Management	Clean and dry
	Skin:
	topical: clotrimazole tds, *continue for 2 weeks after lesions*
	resolved
	oral treatment if resistant
	Scalp: systemic treatment needed
	Also see below

Ringworm

- Use imidazoles.

Nails

- Amorolfine nail lacquer: fingernails: 3–6 months; toenails: 6–12 months (until nail grows out).
- Oral terbinafine: fingernails: 6 weeks; toenails: 3 months.
- 'Pulsed' oral itraconazole: 7 days, repeat after 3 weeks (2 courses for fingernails, 3 for toenails).

Pityriasis versicolor

- Topical: selenium sulphide shampoo used as lotion – leave 30 mins then wash off.
- Oral: fluconazole, itraconazole (**not** terbinafine).

Candidiasis

- *Topical*: clotrimazole.
- *Oral treatment*: fluconazole.
- *Associated angular cholitis*: nystatin ointment.

Scalp

- Systemic treatment usually needed: terbinafine or itraconazole.

Oral candidiasis

- Nystatin or myconazole.

Nappy rash

- Frequent changing nappies, air dry.
- Barrier cream (e.g. Metanium), bath oils, moisturisers.
- Satellite lesions = candidiasis: Timodine cream (= nystatin + hydrocortisone 0.5%).

Pityriasis rosea

- Not fungal, herald patch, pink macules, no treatment needed, fade 4–8 weeks, 1% hydrocortisone for itching.

Terbinafine

- Nails and scalp.

Acne

Data gathering

History	Duration, location
	Effect on self-esteem
	Treatments already tried
	Contraception / pregnancy
	PCOS: weight gain, menstrual irregularity, hirsutism
	Drug history
	Progestogen: e.g. COCP, POP, Mirena coil
Social history	Effect on social life
	Relationships
Red flags	Depression, severe effect on functioning
Examination	Erythema, comedones, pustules, scarring, cysts

Interpersonal skills

ICE	Effect on life, ascertain health beliefs
	Do not dismiss patient's concerns if acne is mild – show empathy
	Hidden request for contraception

Management

Investigations	
Management	Treat early if inflammatory to prevent scarring
	Conservative
	Wash twice daily with mild soap, avoid picking/scratching
	Medical
	Topical: benzoyl peroxide, retinoid creams, topical antibiotics
	Oral antibiotics: e.g. oxytetracycline; inform at least 3–6 months treatment required
	COCP: e.g. Dianette
Safety net	Regular follow up
	Refer for specialist initiation of isotretinoin (Roaccutane)

Myths

- Acne is not caused by poor hygiene or unhealthy diet – too much washing can be detrimental.
- Sunbeds often do not help.
- Medical treatments do work if used correctly.

Eczema

Based on NICE guidelines (2007)

Data gathering

History	Duration, site, itch
	Precipitant: allergen, stress
	Impact on life, sleep and self-esteem
	
	Past medical history / family history
	    Atopy: hayfever, asthma
	Drug history
	    Treatments already tried

Social history	Stress: work, home, relationships Smoking, alcohol Occupation
Red flags	Secondary infection Child: failure to thrive, GI symptoms (consider food allergy)
Examination	Distribution: flexural, seborrhoeic, contact (necklace, watch, belt) Erythema, papules, vesicles, crusting, weeping, dry Lichenification, scarring, excoriation Cushinoid appearance

Interpersonal skills

ICE	Depression screen Empathy with patient's / parent's situation
For patient	*"Sometimes called dermatitis, inflammation of skin, itchy skin condition"* *"Controlled and not cured"* *"Child **may** grow out of it, but it occasionally persists"*

Management

Investigations	Skin prick testing if contact dermatitis and unknown allergen
Management	Avoid allergens, perfumed products, detergents (e.g. gloves when washing up) *Medical* 　　Soap substitute: e.g. aqueous cream, emulsifying ointment 　　Emollients 　　Topical steroids (1% hydrocortisone for face or young 　　　children) *Severe* 　　Wet wrapping over steroids/emollients if severe 　　Phototherapy 　　Immunosuppression: oral steroids, tacrolimus *Infection* 　　Topical: fusidic acid cream (short courses to avoid 　　　resistance) 　　Oral: flucloxacillin, acyclovir (for herpes, refer same day) *Other* 　　Antihistamine for itch (not for routine use)
Safety net	Regular review with compliance assessment Refer if unresponsive / severe or suspicion of occupational or 　herpes infection

- Exclusion diets are controversial and generally only with dietician advice in children.
- Asian and Afro-Carribeans: extensor and discoid subtypes more common.
- Complimentary therapies: no good evidence base, caution against use.

Psoriasis

Data gathering

History	Distribution, duration Joint pain, nails and hair Treatments so far Precipitants: trauma, stress, infections, drugs (lithium, beta blockers, NSAIDs, ACE inhibitors) *Family history*
Social history	Smoking, alcohol Stress: work, home, relationships
Red flags	Erythroderma, widespread pustular psoriasis
Examination	Clinical diagnosis Well-defined scaly silvery-red plaques on extensor surfaces and scalp Koebner phenomenon Nail pitting, arthropathy

Interpersonal skills

ICE	Effect on life, self-esteem
For patient	*"Not infectious/contagious, not curable, can be controlled with treatments"* *"Exact cause unknown, strong familial component"*

Management

Investigations	Skin biopsies if difficult diagnosis (refer)
Management	*Conservative* 　　Support groups, education, avoid stressors, smoking cessation *Medical* 　　Emollients *Inflammatory psoriasis:* topical steroids *Chronic stable plaque psoriasis:* • vitamin D analogues – well tolerated • coal tar • dithranol: stains clothing, irritative to skin, for flexures only *Scalp psoriasis:* emollients, salicylic acid, coal tar, steroid preparations *Refer for:* • PUVA • oral retinoids • immunosuppressants – methotrexate, cyclosporin
Safety net	Regular review Refer if red flags, uncertain diagnosis or uncontrolled

Ear pain

Data gathering

History	Hearing, discharge, bleeding Fever, URTI, swimming Trauma, foreign body Toothache, dental problems
Red flags	Head injury, longstanding symptoms
Examination	Ear Mastoid Temporomandibular joint Skin: shingles, boil/furuncle Cranial nerves: facial nerve

Interpersonal skills

ICE	

Management

Investigations	Swab if discharge

Management	*Acute otitis media*
	    Analgesia, amoxil if persists >48 h
	Eustacian tube dysfunction
	    Regular warm drinks +/– decongestants
	Otitis externa
	    Keep dry, antibiotic ear drops: gentisone, sofradex
	Perforated ear drum
	    Consider amoxicillin 1 weeks, refer if not improving 2–6
	        weeks / (earlier if marginal)
	Boil / furuncle
	    Analgesia +/– I&D
	Temporomandibular joint
	    Analgesia, reassurance, relaxation, dental opinion if
	    persists
	Dental
	    Analgesia, amoxicillin, dentist

Safety net	

Wax: not usually painful, treat with olive oil drops 1–2 weeks, avoid cotton buds.

Tinnitus

Data gathering

History	"What do you mean?" Ringing, buzzing, other noise
	Unilateral vs. bilateral Loud noise exposure Head injury Headache Ear infections

	Meniere's
	    Hearing loss, dizziness, earache / fullness in ear, nausea
	 Depression screen
	    Effect on life, sleep
	 Drug history
	    Loop diuretics, aspirin, NSAIDs

Red flags	Unilateral, head injury, evidence of raised ICP Suicidal ideation: chronic tinnitus is a risk factor
Examination	BP Ears: otitis externa / media, wax Mental state

Interpersonal skills

ICE	Effect on life, depression, stress

Management

Investigations	FBC (anaemia) Audiometry
Management	Reassurance (patients often worried about brain tumour and hypertension) Most self-resolve Tinnitus Masker: available through ENT Support groups: Tinnitus Association Treat co-existing problems: wax, stress, otitis
Safety net	*Refer if:* • persistent • unilateral (acoustic neuroma) • Meniere's (for diagnosis = idiopathic dilation of endolymphatic spaces)

Causes: anaemia, head injury, drugs, noise exposure, acoustic neuroma (unilateral), Meniere's

Dental pain

Data gathering

History	May present as facial, neck or ear pain Fever, swelling, discharge / unusual taste in mouth Previous episodes Is patient registered with dentist?
Social history	Diet, occupation
Red flags	
Examination	Teeth, lymph nodes: tap tooth/gum with tongue depressor to illicit tenderness Examine as appropriate: • ENT, sinuses, salivary glands including parotid • cranial nerves • eyes • skin

Interpersonal skills

ICE	Important to find out patient's ICE early on Effect on life: eating, sleep

Management

Investigations	
Management	Ensure patient understands dental consultation required for proper assessment Analgesia Amoxicillin 5–7 days if suspect abscess or root canal infection
Safety net	Dental review

Labyrinthitis / vestibular neuronitis

Data gathering

History	Light-headed vs. sensation of rotatory movement
	Precipitants: head movements, lying down, stress, trauma
	Recent illness / URTI
	
	Associated symptoms
	    Nausea / vomiting
	    Menniere's: tinnitus, fullness / sensation in ear, reduced
	       hearing
	    Infection: ear, meningitis
	Drug history
	    Aminoglycosides, antihypertensives (especially beta
	       blockers), anti-convulsants

Social history	Driving Alcohol, recreational drugs

Red flags	Neurological symptoms: headache, weakness, sensory
	    disturbance
	Unilateral tinnitus and/or hearing loss: suspect acoustic
	    neuroma

Examination	Should be no abnormalities except maybe some horizontal nystagmus Targeted neurological examination: • cranial nerves • cerebellar signs (DANISH – <u>d</u>ysdiadocokinesis, <u>a</u>taxia, <u>n</u>ystagmus, <u>i</u>ntention tremor, <u>s</u>lurred speech, <u>h</u>ypotonia ENT: • mastoid • Hallpike manoeuvre

Interpersonal skills

ICE	Effect on life, occupation, stress
For patient	*"Viral infection of inner ear that controls balance"*

Management

Investigations	Bloods: FBC, U&Es, TFTs, glucose Audiometry

Management	*Conservative*
	    Reassurance not brain tumour
	    Will get better by itself within a few weeks
	    No driving
	Medical
	    Vestibular suppressants: stemetil, antihistamines,
	        domperidone

Safety net	*Refer if:* • focal neurological features or suspect acoustic neuroma • suspect Meniere's disease • no resolution in 4–6 weeks or rapidly worsening symptoms

Snoring

Data gathering

History	How often?
	Disturbed sleep? Apnoeas? (witness account often required)
	Daytime sleepiness? Irritability?
	Drug history
	Sleeping tablets
Social history	Alcohol, weight gain
Red flags	
Examination	BMI
	Collar size (>17 associated with obstructive sleep apnoea)
	ENT: any obvious obstruction
	Chest, heart, thyroid signs

Interpersonal skills

ICE	Depression screen, effect on partner and relationship with partner
For patient	*"Obstruction can be anywhere from nose to base of tongue"*

Management

Investigations	TFTs
	Sleep studies
Management	Weight loss, exercise, smoking cessation
	Conservative
	Ear plugs for partner
	Nasal dilators
	CPAP (mainly for obstructive sleep apnoea)
	Medical
	Stop alcohol and sedatives
	Surgical
	Nasal surgery: e.g. turbinate reduction, septoplasty, polypectomy
Safety net	Support patient and partner

Painful and red eye

Data gathering

History	General
	How much pain? History of pain
	Visual disturbance, discharge, photophobia
	Contact lenses, spectacles
	Specific questions
	Foreign body, trauma (abrasion)
	Haloes, dusk, nausea / vomiting (glaucoma)
	Reading (long sightedness)
	URTI (conjunctivitis, sinusitis)
	Systemic symptoms (iritis/scleritis/episcleritis)
	Vesicular rash (herpes simplex)
	Itchy, sore, grittiness, precipitant/allergen (conjunctivitis: allergic/infective)
Red flags	Sudden loss of vision
	Temporal arteritis
	Chronic symptoms
Examination	Inspection +/– eversion of eyelid
	Fluoroscein
	Eye movements
	Pupil reflexes
	(Consider visual acuity, fields, fundoscopy)
	+/– take swab
	Temporal arteritis

Interpersonal skills

ICE	

Management

Investigations	
Management	Conjunctivitis: leave or use chloramphenicol or cromoglycate/antihistamines
	Corneal abrasion: review in 2 days, give eyepad if amethocaine / local anaesthetic used

Safety net	Sudden visual loss – refer immediately:
	• temporal arteritis – consider prednisolone 80 mg stat
	• acute angle closure glaucoma – consider pilocarpine 4% drops every 5 mins
	• migraine – consider referral if atypical or unsure of diagnosis

- *Painful and red:* often need referral: glaucoma, herpes simplex, foreign body, abrasion.
- *Painful and not red*: often seen in general practice: stress, refractive error, **beware GCA, retrobulbar neuritis**.
- *Not painful and red:* conjunctivitis, subconjunctival haemorrhage.

Temporal artery + fever = giant cell arteritis / temporal arteritis.
Cloudy cornea and pupil dilation = glaucoma.

Prostate-specific antigen

Patient should decide, after discussion with their doctor, whether to have a PSA test. Important to give written information.

The patient needs to be told the following:
- prostate cancer is but one of several causes of a raised PSA (non-specific test)
- all patients with a significantly raised PSA should have a prostate biopsy
- 1 in 5 men with a normal PSA will have prostate cancer
- 2 in 3 men with a raised PSA will not have cancer
- there is no conclusive evidence that detection of early prostate cancer leads to longer survival
- the test cannot distinguish between aggressive and slow-growing cancers, and may detect tumours that would not otherwise become evident in the patient's lifetime

The test is of most value in patients who are 'high risk', i.e. those > 70 years, Afro-Caribbeans, and those with a family history.

At the time of the test, the patient should not have:
- a UTI
- ejaculated within 48 hours
- a *per rectum* examination within 1 week
- a prostate biopsy within 6 weeks

Age-related PSA reference ranges:
- 50–59 years ≥3.0
- 60–69 years ≥4.0
- >70 years >5.0

Causes of raised PSA:
- acute urinary retention / catheterisation
- BPH/ TURP
- old age
- prostatitis
- prostate carcinoma

Haematuria

Data gathering

History	"Can you see blood in your urine?"
	Painful? Clots? Frothy urine?
	
	Confounders
	    Beetroot, rifampicin
	GU symptoms
	    Irritative/UTI
	    Obstructive
	Past medical history
	    Recent illness / sore throat, kidney stones

Social history	Occupation – chemicals, dyes Smoking, alcohol
Red flags	Weight loss, malaise, anorexia Painless macroscopic haematuria Persistant microscopic haematuria; *"fewer than 1% have cancer"*
Examination	Obtain permission, chaperone BP, abdomen, genitalia, *per rectum*

Interpersonal skills

ICE	

Management

Investigations	Urine dip and MCS Bloods for U&Es if obstructive symptoms
Management	Treat as UTI if painful Analgesia Refer if red flags
Follow up	Repeat urine dip after 1 week

Differential diagnoses: UTI, renal stone, cancer, trauma.

Painless macroscopic haematuria

Refer using 2 week rule.

Renal tract stone

Refer urgently if:
- first presentation
- obstruction on imaging
- very painful
- reduced renal function
- infection

Otherwise:
- fluids, analgesia
- MSU, bloods (FBC, CRP, U&Es, calcium, albumin, phosphate)
- plain abdominal film
- refer outpatients

Erectile dysfunction

Data gathering

History	"*Tell me more about this*"
	"*Are you able to have erections?*"
	"*Difficulty maintaining an erection?*"
	Erections at night or morning? Sexual desire?
	
	Onset
	  Gradual vs. sudden onset
	  Previously sexually active? Previous problems?
	Past medical history
	  CVD: hypertension, DM, raised cholesterol, obesity,
	    peripheral vascular disease
	  Trauma
	Drug history
	  Antihypertensives

Social history	Relationship – ?long term Work, home, finances, other stressors Alcohol, drugs, smoking Exercise
Red flags	Urinary symptoms, prostatism, GI symptoms
Examination	BMI, BP External genitalia – Peyronie's, hypospadius, testicular atrophy *Per rectum* if > 50 years

Interpersonal skills

ICE	Stress, depression and anxiety Occupation, family, finances, sleep

Management

Investigations	Bloods: glucose, cholesterol, U&Es, hormone profile (LH/ FSH, testosterone)

Management	*Conservative*
	     Psychosexual counselling
	 Medical
	     PDE5 inhibitors*
	 Surgical
	     Penile injections, prostheses, vacuum devices

*PDE5 Inhibitors

- Examples are Viagra, Cialis, Levitra.
- Take 1 hour before sex.
- *"Increases blood flow to penis".*

Contraindications:
- nitrates, hypotension
- recent CVA/MI/unstable angina
- caution in sickle cell disease, leukaemia, multiple myeloma (priapism)

NHS scripts can be issued if:
- prostate cancer/radical pelvic surgery – **not TURP**
- pelvic or spinal injury
- DM
- renal failure
- MS, **spina bifida**, Parkinson's Disease, polio, single gene neurological disease

Benign prostatic hyperplasia

Data gathering

History	Irritative
	    Dysuria, frequency, urgency
	Obstructive
	    Hesitancy, poor stream, nocturia
	Infective
	    Fever, urethral discharge, polydipsia, DM
	Others
	    Incontinence, bowel habit, abdominal pain, sexual
	        function

Social history	Fluid intake Caffeine Alcohol
Red flags	Bone pain, haematuria Weight loss, lethargy
Examination	Bladder, kidneys Rectal examination

Interpersonal skills

ICE	Effect on life
For patient	"The prostate is a gland, size of a chestnut, which sits at base of bladder, and surrounds the tube through which urine passes"

Management

Investigations	Urine – dip, MSU Bloods – U&Es, PSA, glucose, Ca Trans-rectal USS prostate X-ray pelvis/hips – ?metastases

Management	*Conservative*
	    Avoid evening fluids
	    Decrease caffeine and alcohol
	    Bladder retraining
	    Avoid constipation
	Medical
	    Alpha-blocker (relaxes smooth muscle) – warn postural
	       hypotension
	    Finasteride – shrinks prostate, can take 6 months to work
	Surgical
	    TURP
	Alternative
	    Saw Palmetto – can be effective!

Safety net	Refer if: • raised U&Es • ?cancer – haematuria, abnormal PR, weight loss... • treatment resistant • urinary retention **Think**: could urinary symptoms be due to diabetes?

Urinary incontinence

Data gathering

History	*Stress incontinence*: coughing, sneezing, laughing
	Urge incontinence: frequency day and night, urge
	Obstructive incontinence: hesitancy, poor stream/dribbling, nocturia, incomplete emptying
	Passive incontinence: passing urine without realising
	UTI: dysuria, fever
	Fluids: evening, caffeine, alcohol
	
	Past medical history
	    CVA, spinal problems, obstetrics, surgery
	Drug history
	    Diuretics, TCAs

Red flags	?Prostate cancer in men
Examination	Abdomen, *per vagina, per rectum*, external genitalia Bladder, kidney Enlarged prostate, constipation Pelvic masses, vaginitis Inguinal herniae

Interpersonal skills

ICE	Effect on life and self esteem, embarrassment

Management

Investigations	Urine dip and MCS U&Es, glucose Urinary diary

Management	Support
	District nurse – incontinence pads, catheters
	
	Stress incontinence
	    Stop smoking and drinking alcohol and caffeine
	    Weight loss, avoid constipation
	    Pelvic floor exercises +/– physiotherapy
	    Prolapse: ring pessary, surgery
	Urge incontinence
	    Bladder retraining – less frequent urination
	    Oxybutinin 2.5–5 mg bd
	    Tolterodine 1–2 mg bd

Safety net	Refer if: • not responding to treatment • unsure of diagnosis • surgery is needed – urodynamic studies • ?prostate cancer

Testicular pain

Data gathering

History	Trauma Recent illness (mumps), fever GU symptoms: irritative (frequency, urgency, dysuria) GI symptoms: abdominal pain, vomiting, bowel habit Sexual history if ?STI-related
Red flags	Cancer: weight loss, anorexia, lethargy Torsion
Examination	Abdomen, penis/scrotum +/– transillumination

Interpersonal skills

ICE	Chaperone?

Management

Management	Analgesia, wait and see Epididymitis: urethral swab (gonorrhoea, chlamydia) Urine dip / MSU Ciprofloxacin +/– GU clinic referral
Safety net	Refer immediately if very painful/torsion Refer using 2 week rule if ?cancer

Consider differential diagnosis: renal colic, hernia, groin strain.

Chronic kidney disease

Data gathering

History	Fatigue, malaise
	GI: anorexia, nausea, vomiting *GU*: nocturia, polyuria *CCF*: SOB, ankle swelling

	Past medical history / family history
	    Hypertension, CVD, DM, UTI, connective tissue diseases,
	      cancer
	    Renal disease
	Drug history
	    NSAIDs, ACE inhibitors, diuretics, lithium

Social history	Smoking, alcohol Support
Red flags	Rapid deterioration in renal function (acute renal failure) Newly diagnosed renal dysfunction (assume this is acute renal failure until proven otherwise) Nephrotic syndrome Malignant hypertension Hyperkalaemia
Examination	BP, weight, fever Anaemia, uraemia CCF Palpable bladder Signs of underlying cause

Interpersonal skills

ICE	Effect on life

Management

Investigations	Urine dipstick (blood, protein) Urine MCS for casts FBC, U&Es, estimated GFR, LFTs, cholesterol, calcium, phosphate, bicarbonate, glucose Hepatitis screen, rheumatolgy screen, HIV USS renal tract (also CT/MRI, renal biopsy in secondary care)

Management	Conservative
	Smoking cessation, weight loss, exercise
	Low salt and low alcohol diet
	Medical
	Tight control of blood pressure
	Avoid NSAIDs and nephrotoxic drugs
	ACE inhibitor if microalbuminuria (monitor U&Es and potassium)
Safety net	Monitor U&Es, CVD risk (BP, cholesterol)
	Urgent referral if red flags

Management of CKD in primary care

Based on the guidelines of The Renal Association

CKD stage	GFR (ml/min)	Test frequency	Management
I	>90	12 monthly	Normal if no other evidence of kidney damage*
II	60–90	12 monthly	Normal if no other evidence of kidney damage*
III	30–60	6–12 monthly	Routinely refer if: • progressively worsening renal functioning • anaemia • electrolyte imbalance • microscopic haematuria or elevated protein:creatinine ratio • uncontrolled BP • systemic illness suspected, e.g. SLE Check parathyroid hormone at diagnosis (if raised check vitamin D levels, refer if still raised despite adequate vitamin D replacement) Immunisation: influenza, pneumococcus
IV	15–30	3–6 monthly	Urgent referral (routine if known stable CKD IV) 3-monthly U&Es, FBC, calcium, phosphate, bicarbonate, parathyroid hormone Immunisation: hepatitis B
V	<15	3 monthly	Immediate referral

*Patients with no evidence of kidney damage and GFR >60 ml/min are assumed not to have CKD.

Evidence of chronic kidney damage

• Persistent microalbuminuria, proteinuria, haematuria (exclude urological causes).
• Structural abnormalities of the kidney.
• Glomerulonephritis on biopsy.

Proteinuria

- Exclude UTI.
- Confirm with early morning urine sample sent to laboratory (to exclude postural proteinuria).
- Persistent proteinuria – at least 2 tests, 1–2 weeks apart.
- Refer to nephrology if:
  - urine protein:creatinine ratio >100 mg/mmol
  - reduced GFR

Haematuria

- Exclude infection, trauma and menstruation.
- No need for laboratory confirmation.
- Check U&Es and for proteinuria.
- Refer to urology if: macroscopic or microscopic and >50 years.
- Refer to nephrology if: microscopic with proteinuria or <50 years.

Refer for investigation for renal artery stenosis

- BP >150/90 despite three anti-hypertensive agents.
- Recurrent pulmonary oedema despite normal echo.
- Rising serum creatinine with raised CVD risk.
- Unexplained hypokalaemia with hypertension.

Menorrhagia

Data gathering

History	How much blood?
	• number of towels, soaked through, flooding
	• clots
	• days of bleeding
	When did heavy periods start?
	Sudden change?
	Associated symptoms
	Painful periods, pelvic pain/pressure
	Thyroid disturbance
	Anaemia
	SOB, fatigue
	Gynaecology history
	Periods – regular, IMB, PCB, LMP
	Smear
	Sexual activity + STI risk/discharge
	Contraception
	Obstetric history
	Past medical history / family history
	Bleeding disorders
	Drug history
	Aspirin
Social history	
Red flags	>40 years, sudden onset
	Organic cause: IMB, PCB, pelvic mass, PID
Examination	Chaperone, permission
	Consider pelvic examination

Interpersonal skills

ICE	Treatments already tried, effect on life

Management

Investigations	All women should have FBC
	TFTs if symptomatic
	Coagulation screen if since menarche +/– family history
	FSH if menopausal
	STI screen if at risk of infection
	Ultrasound scan if there is a possibility of a structural abnormality
Management	*Conservative*
	Menstrual diary
	Medical
	Tranexamic acid: 1–1.5 g tds–qds at start of heavy bleeding for 5 days
	Mefanamic acid: 250–500 mg tds (better for pain)
	COCP
	Norethisterone: 10 mg tds stops torrential bleeds after 2 days, then 5 mg bd for 12 days
	Surgical
	Mirena IUS (NICE 1st line), especially if contraception needed
	Transcervical resection of endometrium, endometrial laser abalation, hysterectomy
Safety net	Refer if red flags

Amenorrhoea/ oligomenorrhoea

Data gathering

History	Primary
	    Menarche
	    Genetic
	Secondary (usually hormonal)
	    Weight loss
	    Stress / depression / eating disorders / exercise
	
	Pregnancy: LMP, sexual activity, wanting to become pregnant?
	Prolactin: galactorrhoea
	PCOS: hirsutism, acne, weight gain
	Menopause: hot flushes, mood change, concentration
	Hypo/hyperthyroidism / Cushing's: lethargy, skin changes
	
	Drug history
	    COCP, steroids

Social history	
Red flags	Pelvic mass
Examination	Secondary sexual characteristics BP, weight Gynae: smear, bimanual, speculum Pelvic ultrasound scan rather than examination if young girl

Interpersonal skills

ICE	Chaperone Effect on life

Management

Investigations	Rule out pregnancy FSH/LH, testosterone, prolactin TFTs, glucose Pelvic ultrasound scan
Management	If normal – reassurance If patient wanting to get pregnant – refer for ?clomiphene
Safety net	Refer as per cause

- Primary amenorrhoea = no periods by 16 years of age, refer to gynaecology.
- Beware girl who has recently stopped COCP – wait 3–6 months.

Premenstrual tension

Data gathering

History	Effect on life Periods, bleeding, smear, contraception, obstetric history
Social history	Smoking, alcohol
Red flags	
Examination	

Interpersonal skills

ICE	Depression, anxiety, stressors, effect on life

Management

Investigations	

Management	Support, reassurance
	3 months menstrual diary
	
	Conservative
	    Exercise – menstrual diary
	    Diet
	    Stop smoking, healthy lifestyle, alcohol
	    Relaxation
	Medical
	    Evening primrose oil
	    Vitamin B6 from day 14 to menses
	    Calcium supplements for breast tenderness, headaches, cramps
	    NSAIDs
	    COCP
	    Luteal progesterone
	    SSRIs

Safety net	

Polycystic ovary syndrome

Data gathering

Presentation	Weight gain Acne Difficulty in conceiving
History	*"Any unusual hair growth?"* Periods, oligomenorrhoea, LMP *"Are you trying to become pregnant?"* Obs and gynae history
Social history	Smoking
Red flags	
Examination	BP, weight Acne, hirsutism

Interpersonal skills

ICE	Fertility, appearance /self esteem
For patient	*"Cause is unknown"* *"Common: 1 in 10–20 women have varying degrees of this"*

Management

Investigations	Raised LH and testosterone Glucose, cholesterol Ultrasound scan for polycystic ovaries

Management	*Conservative*
	    Reassure that it is a common condition
	    Weight loss, diet, exercise
	    Smoking cessation
	    Contraception
	Medical
	    COCP if not wanting pregnancy
	    Metformin – helps ovulation, oligomenorrhoea
	Fertility: clomiphene – if wanting child (refer to gynaecology,
	    high success rates)
	
	Treat hirsutism and acne

Safety net	

Hirsutism

Data gathering

History	Recent onset vs. longstanding

	PCOS
	    Periods, acne, weight gain, fertility
	Family history
	    Ethnic origin
	Drug history
	    Phenytoin, steroids, cyclosporin

Red flags	Galactorrhoea, recent onset/rapidly worsening Pelvic mass Virilisation
Examination	Weight, BMI, BP Hair pattern, acne Bimanual vaginal examination – if suspect ovarian/androgen secreting tumour

Interpersonal skills

ICE	Effect on life

Management

Investigations	Not needed if longstanding and regular periods Testosterone, LH, FSH

Management	Weight loss if overweight
	Cosmetic: bleaching, shaving, waxing, hair-removal creams, electrolysis
	
	Medical
	    Dianette – establish risk of CVD and DVT/PE first (smoking, weight, family history, etc.)
	    Eflornithine cream (Vaniqa) – only if other drugs not working

Safety net	Refer if red flags

- Hirsutism = *male-pattern* excess hair.
- Affects 1 in 10 women.
- Most is familial.
- Distinguish early on in the consultation if recent or longstanding.

Combined oral contraceptive pill

Stopping ovulation is the main mechanism of action; it also thickens cervical mucus and causes endometrial changes.

Disadvantages	Advantages
1.2 x relative risk of breast cancer	50% reduction in ovarian + uterine cancer
DVT (15–30/100 000 compared to 5/100 000 background or 60/100 000 pregnant)	
5% develop hypertension after 5 years Smoking gives 3-times increased risk of vascular disease	No known increased MI risk

Absolute CI	Relative CI (don't give if more than one present)
DVT Heart disease / hypertension / hypercholesterolaemia Focal migraine with aura Cancer of breast/cervix Sickle cell disease	Family history of arterial disease, DVT DM, hypertension, smoking, weight, age >35 years, migraine

Side effects

Breakthrough bleeding – settles by 3 months.
Nausea, breast tenderness, bloating, PMT, mood change, vaginal discharge.

Examination

Weight, BP, smear status.

Management

Start day 1–5 of menstrual cycle, no extra precautions needed.

Follow up

At 3 months, then 6–12 months.
Check smoking, BP, weight, smear status, new risk factors.

Breakthrough bleeding

Causes: STI, enzyme inducers, pregnancy, compliance/vomiting, cervical lesions.
Management:
- investigate after 3 months – examine, swabs, consider ultrasound scan
- try pill with different progesterone or higher oestrogen

No withdrawal bleed

Consider pregnancy, change to lower progesterone COCP.

Stopping pill to conceive

Ideally use condoms for 3 months until normal period passed.

Emergency contraception

Data gathering

History	*"Why do you need the morning after pill?"*
	When had unprotected sex? Any other times had sex? With whom?
	Consensual sex?
	
	Contraception
	    What do you normally use for contraception?
	    Why failed? How many missed pills?
	Contraindications
	    History of pelvic infections
	    Ectopic pregnancies
	Past medical history
	    Valvular heart disease
	Drug history
	STI risk
	    Regular partner?

Social history	STI risk
Red flags	STI, ?pregnant/LMP Rape or vulnerable adult
Examination	BP, weight

Interpersonal skills

ICE	*"How important is it that you do not become pregnant?"*

Management

Investigations	
Management	*"No contraceptive is 100% effective"* Morning after pill Copper IUD

Safety net	*"You should have a pregnancy test if your next period is abnormally light or delayed"* *"Return promptly if any lower abdominal pain"* *"Barrier contraception needed until next period"* Long term contraception STI risk/screen Smears up to date Vulnerability

Levonorgestrel 1.5 mg single dose (Levonelle)

- Licensed up to 72 hours.
- Inform patient *"effectiveness rapidly decreases with delay in using it"*.
- If vomit within 2 hours, take another dose (<1 in 20 women).
- May have some light bleeding or spotting.

Copper-containing IUD = most effective method

- *"Small device which contains copper put into your womb"*.
- Effective up to 5 days, or 5 days after ovulation.
- Take swabs.
- Antibiotic cover.

Contraindications:
- Pregnancy, severe anaemia, immunosuppression.
- Recent STI, PID.
- Unexplained PV bleeding.
- Genital malignancy.
- Copper – copper allergy, Wilson's.

Termination of pregnancy request

Data gathering

History	How did you find out you were pregnant? Were you using contraception at the time? (split condom/ missed pill) With regular partner? Does he know you are pregnant? Was sex consensual? *Social context* Why do you want an abortion? Have you spoken to anyone else about this? *Date pregnancy* LMP? Normal period? *Past medical history* Gynae/obs, psychiatric history
Social history	Home, work, children, relationships
Red flags	Socially isolated, domestic violence, abuse
Examination	BP, BMI

Interpersonal skills

ICE	Ensure patient makes best decision for her and is well supported

Management

Investigations	Pregnancy test
Management	*"Are you aware of your options?"* *"How sure are you that you want an abortion?"* Obliged to go though some options with patient before proceeding: • have baby • adoption • TOP – medical/surgical
Safety net	Long term contraception / STI screen Psychological and emotional support

Complications of termination

- Infection – 5%, minimised by antibiotics and pre-procedure screening.
- Cervical trauma – 1%, less risk in early termination.
- Rare: haemorrhage (1.5/1000), perforation of uterus (1–4/1000), failed termination (2–5/1000).
- No evidence to link termination with subsequent infertility or pre-term delivery.

Psychological effects

- Only long term in small proportion.
- Early distress is common – usually a continuation of the symptoms present before abortion.
- Remember negative effects on both the mother and the child where abortion has been denied.

At under 7 weeks' gestation

Medical abortion, e.g. Mifepristone orally followed after 48 h by Gemeprost vaginally. Avoid suction termination.

At 7–15 weeks' gestation

- Conventional suction termination is appropriate. Local or general anaesthesia.
- Medical abortion may be preferable above 12 weeks.

Terminations at >15 weeks' gestation

Dilatation and evacuation, preceded by preparation or medical abortion.

Subfertility

Data gathering

History	How long trying to conceive? Without contraception? How often having sex? Any problems with sex?
	Either partner had a child? Previous pregnancies? Miscarriage? TOP?
	Regular cycles
	Past medical history General health, STI risk *Female*: surgery including appendectomy, rubella vaccination *Male*: testicular trauma, mumps, varicocoele *Drug history* NSAIDs may impair fertility, antipsychotics, teratogens
Social history	Smoking, alcohol, recreational drugs Stress
Red flags	STI, chronic disease, pelvic pathology, ambiguous genitalia
Examination	*Female* BMI, BP, hitsutism / androgenisation Abnormal genitalia, pelvic mass *Male* Gynacomastia, abnormal genitalia, inguinal hernia, testicles

Interpersonal skills

ICE	Preferably joint consultation with both partners; important to investigate both partners Difficult to cover all in single consultation, may need to schedule another consultation
For patient	*"Subfertility affects 1 in 6 couples"*

Management

Investigations	Female
	STI screen
	LH, FSH, luteal progesterone, prolactin, TFTs
	Transvaginal ultrasound
	Male
	Semen analysis
Management	Reassurance: "*90% of healthy couples conceive within 12 months*"
	Conservative
	Pre-conception advice – folic acid, smoking cessation, alcohol, weight, diet, etc.
	Sexual intercourse 2–3 times a week
	Medical
	Clomiphene
	Surgical
	In-vitro fertilisation, intracytoplasmic sperm injection
Safety net	Refer as per local criteria to assisted conception unit or equivalent, e.g. typically:
	• no conception after 18 months
	• woman between 35 and 40 years of age with no living child
	Abnormal investigations – refer as per cause

Screening
Cervical screening

To *prevent* cancer (not cure it; detects pre-cancerous lesions):
- 25–64 years of age: 3-yearly for 25–49 year-olds, 5-yearly for 50-64 year-olds
- >65 years if previous abnormal smear or no smear since 50 years

2000 new cases cervical cancer/year, most of these women have not had recent smear.
- 1 in 20 are borderline, very few develop cancer
- 1 in 20 are mild dyskaryosis, cancer very unlikely
- 1 in 100 are moderate dyskaryosis, pre-cancerous, intermediate probability of developing cancer

Screening result	Action
Negative	Inform patient, routine recall
Inadequate	Repeat as soon as possible (definitely within 3 months) Refer colposcopy if three consecutive inadequate smears
Borderline	Endocervical cells: refer colposcopy Squamous cells: • repeat within 6 months • three consecutive negatives 6 months apart before routine recall
Mild dyskaryosis	Ideally refer colposcopy Can repeat in 6 months – if negative, need three negatives 6 months apart before routine recall
Moderate/severe dyskaryosis	Refer colposcopy

Colposcopy

"A more detailed examination of the cervix."
- The doctor uses a speculum and magnifier (colposcope).
- A liquid is used to 'paint' the cervix which shows up the abnormal cells.
- Takes 10–15 mins.
- Biopsy often taken.

Treatments can be undertaken – cryotherapy, laser treatment, loop diathermy.
- Few weeks for the cervix to heal after treatment.
- Once it has healed, a normal sex life can be resumed.
- Does not affect fertility.

Breast cancer screening

50–64 year olds, 3 yearly mammograms (available to patients >65 years on request).

Diagnosing menopause

Defined as no periods for 2 years in those patients <50 years or 1 year for patients >50 years.

Data gathering

History	Bleeding pattern, LMP
	
	Symptoms
	    Flushes/sweats
	    Vaginal dryness, urinary incontinence
	    Anxiety, depression
	Gynae history
	    Smears, mammograms, contraception

Social history	Smoking, alcohol
Red flags	Abnormal bleeding: irregular, painful, PCB, bleeding 1 year after LMP
Examination	BP, weight, breasts

Interpersonal skills

ICE	Depression, anxiety, effect on life

Management

Investigations	?Pregnancy test ?TFTs FSH if uncertain of diagnosis: e.g. <45 years, hysterectomy, on HRT/COCP/POP/IUS
Management	Check patient's understanding Stressors Discuss HRT Other measures to cope with symptoms
Safety net	Should investigate: • irregular or painful bleeding/PCB • bleeding 1 year after LMP

- *Flushes and sweats:* deep breathing exercises, cool environment, evening primrose oil.
- *Topical oestrogens:* help vaginal dryness and reduce UTIs.

Starting hormone replacement therapy

Why start?	Control menopausal symptoms Osteoporosis prevention if <50 years (e.g. hysterectomised)
Risk factors	Smoking Past medical history or family history of breast cancer and PE/DVT Mammograms not up to date
Contraindications	Breast or endometrial cancer DVT/PE Severe liver/kidney/gallbladder disease Otosclerosis (may worsen on HRT)
Side effects	Spotting for first 3 months Fluid retention, breast enlargement

Advantages	Disadvantages
Controls symptoms Prevents osteoporosis and colon cancer Decreases UTIs	Small increase in breast cancer, PE/DVT and stroke • 6/1000 extra cases breast cancer after 5 years • excess risk disappears 5 years after stopping • no increased risk of breast cancer if <50 years

Cyclical	Non-cyclical
Normally start with cyclical preparartions Start on 1st 5 days of cycle For women with periods Perimenopausal women	Women without periods (for at least 1 year) Hysterectomised Been on cyclical for several years and wish to stop periods Tibolone is non-cyclical, less breast cancer risk

• Women without uterus can have oestrogen alone (less risk of breast cancer).

- Tibolone: for women who cannot take oestrogens, protects against osteoporosis, helps symptoms.
- Do not use topical oestrogens for more than 1 year at a time (need more data).
- Can give HRT as patch or implant.
- Can give low dose COCP in fit non-smokers to relieve symptoms of menopause.
- HRT is not contraception.

Follow up

- Every 3 months initially, then every 6–12 months.
- Ask about abnormal bleeding.
- Some women have no bleeds on continuous preps – this can be normal, exclude pregnancy.
- Most women only need up to 5 years of HRT.
- Examination: BP, weight, smears, mammograms.

Antenatal counselling

Assessment of gestational age should be based on an early ultrasound scan rather than the last menstrual period.

Folic acid	400 µg of folic acid up to 12 weeks to reduce neural tube defects 5 mg if high risk suggested by past medical history or family history (coeliac, DM, sickle cell disease, anticonvulsants)
Rubella	Immunisation if needed
Nutrition	Normal diet, five portions of fruit and vegetables per day Drinking plenty of milk to raise stores of vitamins, iron and calcium is reasonable Avoid: • uncooked meat, fish and eggs (toxoplasmosis) • liver (vitamin A) • milk that has not been pasteurised • soft cheeses (listeria) • all fruit and vegetables should be washed (toxoplasmosis) • herbal preparations, caffeine
Exercise	Gentle programme of regular exercise if not already, avoid high impact/contact sports Avoid excessive heating, hot tubs/saunas, scuba diving (birth defects, decompression)
Drug history	As few medicines as possible
Smoking	Avoid, NRT safer than smoking (lower dose nicotine) (Zyban/Champix are contraindicated in pregnancy)
Alcohol	Avoid (1–2 drinks twice a week unlikely to be harmful)
Social history	Maternity rights and benefits Reassure patient it is safe to continue working Check occupation for exposure to harmful agents

Gastro-intestinal symptoms during pregnancy

- Nausea and vomiting of pregnancy generally resolves by 16–20 weeks gestation; ginger and P6 acupressure may be beneficial. Antihistamines have also been used.
- Heartburn – small regular meals, raising the head of bed, antacids.

Illicit drug use

- A multidisciplinary approach is essential.
- Urged to enter detoxification programme before conception or at least stabilised on methadone.
- HIV, Hep B and C screening

Travel

- ?Increased risk of DVT if flying.
- Compression hosiery.
- Also discuss vaccinations and travel insurance if travelling abroad.
- Car seat belts above and below bump rather than over it.

Down syndrome

- 1 in 1000 births; maternal age 30 years 1 in 500, 35 years 1 in 250, 40 years 1 in 60.
- Nuchal scan: 10–13 weeks.
- Triple test: alpha fetoprotein, HCG, estriol at 15–20 weeks.
- Chorionic villus sampling: 8–12 weeks, allows 1st trimester TOP, 1–2% miscarriage rate.
- Amniocentesis: at 15–16 weeks, TOP before 20 weeks, alpha fetoprotein takes 1 week, karyotype 3 weeks, 1% miscarriage rate.

Booking visit

Data gathering

History	How know you are pregnant? LMP + calculate expected due date *Patient and partner* Age, occupation, race *Past medical history, family history, obs and gynae history*
Social history	Alcohol, smoking Social support, finances, home/work
Red flags	Family history, complex past medical / obstetric history
Examination	Weight, BP Heart, chest, abdomen, legs (varicose veins) No need for vaginal examination

Interpersonal skills

ICE	Effect on life

Management

Investigations	Urine: dip + MSU Bloods: FBC, ABO, Hep B, syphillis, HIV, +/– rubella status, haemoglobinopathies
Management	*"Do you have any ideas of how you want to proceed from here?"* *Care*: shared/community/hospital *Diet:* e.g. folic acid *Screening:* e.g. ultrasound scan at 12 and 20 weeks *Benefits:* free prescription and dental care for pregnancy and 12 months after
Safety net	Monthly until 32 weeks, 2-weekly until 36 weeks, weekly after 36 weeks Ultrasound scan, midwives Refer if complex case

Subsequent antenatal visits

Data gathering

History	General health, problems, gestational age
Social history	
Red flags	Bleeding, pain, mood, support
Examination	BP + urine dip Fundal height Fetus: • movements/heart from 12 weeks • presentation from 32 weeks

Interpersonal skills

ICE	Effect on life

Management

Investigations	Screening tests ABO and haemoglobin at 28 and 32 weeks

Paediatrics – general approach

Data gathering

History	Past medical history
	Birth history
	Immunisations
	Developmental history
	Feeding/diet
	Family history
	Drug history
Social history	Family and siblings
	School
Red flags	Developmental delay, poor growth/weight gain
	Child protection issues, abuse/neglect
Examination	Plot on centile charts: height, weight, head circumference
	Alert, responsiveness, hydration

Interpersonal skills

ICE	Concerns, empathy, effect on parents
	Watch out for postnatal depression

ADHD

Data gathering

History	Three main features for at least 6 months in two different situations (e.g. school and home): 1. inattention 2. hyperactivity 3. impulsiveness Above must be abnormal for child's age Normal developmental milestones?
Social history	How is child getting along at school? Friends? Relationships within family Interests and activities
Red flags	Abnormal development Child protection issues
Examination	Height, weight, behaviour and interaction

Interpersonal skills

ICE	Ensure child meets ADHD criteria Empathy

Management

Investigations	
Management	Support and involve entire family in management Family therapy Avoid caffeine and sugary foods/drinks Ignore bad behaviour, reward good behaviour
Safety net	Refer for assessment if meets criteria for ADHD Regular review and support to family

Nocturnal enuresis

Data gathering

History	*Primary vs. secondary*
	    Has child ever been dry?
	    Wet during day?
	    Heavy sleeper
	Gastro-intestinal symptoms
	    Bowel habit
	Family history
	    Bed wetting
	    Siblings

Social history	Family and school
Red flags	Poor growth and development, behavioural problems, neurological symptoms
Examination	Growth Abdomen Spine – sacral dimple/naevus/hair Ankle jerks

Interpersonal skills

ICE	
For patient	*"Delay in maturation of control mechanisms"*

Management

Investigations	Urine dip and MCS

Management	Involve parent and child, and health visitor/school nurse
	
	Advice
	    Avoid evening drinks
	    Lift child to lavatory when parents go to bed
	    Star chart for dry nights
	    +/− nappies/starter pants if <7 years
	Treatment (>7 years only)
	    Enuresis alarm – most respond by 2–3 months, stop after 28 dry nights
	    Desmopressin po/sl (not intranasal) at night, e.g. social occasions

Safety net	Support and follow up

- Specific treatment not needed <7 years.
- Daytime wetting should stop by 4 years of age (refer to urology for neuropathic bladder).
- 10% of 5 year olds still wet bed.

- Reward wanted behaviour.
- Ignore wet nights, no punishment.
- Give a treat if seven consecutive dry nights.

- Secondary nocturnal enuresis = dry for 6 months beforehand.

Depression

Data gathering

Screening questions	Over the past month have you: • felt down, depressed or hopeless? • had little interest or pleasure in doing things?

Biological features	Unintentional weight loss?
	"How has your appetite been?"
	"Are you sleeping well?"
	"How has this affected your day-to-day life?" (this question often brings out the other symptoms: poor concentration, loss energy, hopelessness, thoughts of harm)
	
	Past medical history / family history
	    Depression, mania, DSH / suicide attempts, post-natal depression
	
	Drug history
	    Benzodiazepines, sedatives, St John's Wort, COCP

Social history	Smoking, alcohol, recreational drugs Work, home, relationships, family, finances Children Social support
Red flags	Risk to self – DSH, suicide Risk to others Alternate diagnosis: hypothyroidism, anxiety, grief, PTSD, BPAD, schizophrenia
Examination	Tearfulness, *"hearing voices?"*

Interpersonal skills

ICE	Effect on life Open questions, active listening, empathy Important to involve patient in management plan

Management

Investigations	Consider bloods – TFTs (especially if no stressor)

Management	*Conservative*
	     Support – family, friends, GP, counselling
	     Exercise, diet, stopping drugs / alcohol, watchful waiting
	     Psychology / CBT
	Medical
	     Antidepressants, sleeping tablets (assess risk of overdose first)
	Social
	     Benefits, sick note, social support, child protection issues

Safety net	Refer if high risk / drug use / uncertain diagnosis Follow up in 1 week for most initial cases, negotiate with patient Try to defer antidepressants until next appointment

When to screen for depression

- Chronic disease, carer, life event (death, divorce, pregnancy...), drugs / alcohol, past history.

Antidepressants

- *"These take 2–4 weeks to work, and they are not addictive".*
- *"Need to continue for 6 months after feeling better; do not suddenly stop them".*

Postnatal depression

- Affects up to 12% of women.
- Consider using Edinburgh Postnatal Depression Scale.
- Treat as for normal depression.
- Lower threshold for non-drug treatments when patient is breastfeeding.
- Tricyclics better for breastfeeding women as more data and less secreted in breast milk.
- Be aware of child protection issues.

Anxiety

Based on ICD-10 criteria and NICE guidelines (2007)

Data gathering

Symptoms	Clarify symptoms, e.g. apprehension, irritability, poor sleep, avoidance behaviour When did symptoms first start? Significant events – family, work, finances *Panic disorder* – recurrent episodes, severe anxiety, unpredictable *GAD* – symptoms most of the time *Phobia* – in response to certain well defined situations that are not currently dangerous *Others* – depression, hyperthyroidism
Social history	Caffeine, nicotine, alcohol, recreational drugs Social support networks Occupation
Red flags	Risk to self and/or others
Examination	Mental state BP, pulse, heart

Interpersonal skills

ICE	Effect on daily functioning and occupation Depression can often co-exist
For patient	Inform patient that condition is treatable Support groups and shared decision-making improves outcome

Management

Investigations	Urine – catecholamines Bloods – TFTs, glucose ECG

Management	*Conservative*
	Exercise, relaxation techniques
	Avoid caffeine
	Psychological
	CBT for 1–4 months (longest lasting effect of all treatments – NICE)
	Self-help – computer-aided or bibliotherapy (CBT-based)
	Medical
	SSRI
Safety net	Refer to specialist if two interventions have no significant effect
	Monitor effect with self-complete questionnaires if possible

SSRI

- For example, paroxetine, for at least 6 months, then stop over 4–6 months.
- Warn the patient regarding initial worsening symptoms, delay in effect, and potential withdrawal symptoms if suddenly stopped.
- Can try another SSRI if 1st doesn't work after 12 weeks.

Immediate management
Based on NICE primary care guidelines

- Benzodiazepines – for no longer than 2–4 weeks.
- Sedative antihistamines can also be used.
- Propranolol.

Psychiatric risk assessment

Remember, risk of suicide is different to risk of deliberate self-harm, e.g. a patient may have thoughts of harming themselves without suicidal ideation.

1. Risk of suicide
- Thoughts of harm to self.
- Previous suicide attempts.
- Planned vs. impulsive.

2. Risk of deliberate self harm
- Thoughts of harming self.
- History of harming self.

3. Risk to others
- Thoughts of harming others.
- History of harming others.
- Forensic history.

You may need to work up to asking about suicidal ideas:
- *"How do you feel about the future?"*
- *"Do you feel that life is worth living?"*
- *"Do you have negative thoughts?"*
- *"Have you any thoughts of ending it all?"*
- *"Have you made any plans to end you life/kill yourself?"*

Suicide risk:
- *"Do you think you would try to end your life / kill yourself?"*
- *"What is stopping you?"*
- *"What will you do if you feel suicidal?"*

Also ask about alcohol, recreational drugs, and past psychiatric history.

Recent non-accidental overdose

Data gathering

History	*"Tell me how it happened?"* *"Did you make any plans so you wouldn't be found?"* *"Did you write a suicide note or will"* *"How long have you been feeling this way for?"* *Motivation* 　　*"Why did you do it?"* 　　*"Was there anything that happened that made you do it?"* 　　*"Was this something you planned to do?"* 　　*"How did you feel:* 　　　　• *before you did it?"* 　　　　• *when you were doing it?"* *Risk to self* 　　Impulsive vs. premeditated 　　Cry for help vs. serious intent 　　*"How do you feel about it now?"* 　　*"Do you still think of harming yourself?"* 　　*"What is stopping you from harming yourself now?"* 　　*"What will you do if you feel this way again?"* 　　*"Have you ever tried to harm or kill yourself before?"* *Psychiatric history* 　　History of mental illness – depression, schizophrenia 　　Previous attempts at suicide / self harm
Social history	Social support network – *"Is there anyone you can turn to for support?"* Work, home, relationships, finances Smoking, alcohol, recreational drugs Child protection issues
Red flags	Risk of harm to self / others, psychiatric illness Drug abuse, poor social support Immediate risk of overdose
Examination	Mental state

Interpersonal skills

ICE	Expectations, e.g. sick note, referral, support group

Management

Investigations	Risk assessment
Management	Refer if high risk Support groups – AA, substance misuse
Safety net	Review in 1 week if low risk and no medical problems *"What do you feel needs to happen for you to feel in control of your life again?"* *"What would you do if you felt this way again?"*

Alcoholism

Data gathering

History	Binge vs. daily
	Social vs. alone
	CAGE
	    Need to **C**ut down?
	    Annoyed at criticism to cut down?
	    Guilty about drinking?
	    Eye opener – need an early morning drink?

Social history	Driving
Red flags	Memory, blackouts, functioning, injuries Depression, stress, suicide risk
Examination	BP, weight, Tremor, speech Hands, pulse, jaundice, anaemia, heart, abdomen Neuropathy, encephalopathy

Interpersonal skills

ICE	Effect on life
For patient	Explain risks of alcohol (see below)

Management

Investigations	Bloods – FBC (macrocytosis), LFT, gamma-GT Urine – toxicology screen

Management	*Conservative*
	    Emphasise stopping drinking is patient's responsibility
	    Alcohol diary, Alcoholics Anonymous, support to patient
	      and family
	    Inform DVLA
	Medical
	    Vitamin B and C
	    Consider detoxification (see below)
	Other
	    Treat depression

Safety net	Regular review Admit delirium tremens, haematemesis, pancreatitis

Alcohol detoxification

- Motivation to stop – emphasise patient is responsible for detox success.
- Detox in community over 1 week with chlordiazepoxide, daily dispensing from pharmacy.
- Refer for detox if:
  - delirium tremens / seizures
  - drug user
  - lack of social support

Units

1 unit = ½ pint beer, 25 ml spirits, 125 ml wine

Bottle of wine = 9 units

Recommended intake: men <21, women <14 units/week

Risks of alcohol

- *"It affects every organ in body".*
- Injuries.
- Erectile dysfunction, infertility.
- Brain damage, depression.
- Obesity, diabetes, heart disease.
- Liver damage.
- Cancer: breast, mouth, oesophagus, liver.

Delirium tremens

- Onset is 2–3 days after patient stops drinking.
- Fever, tachycardia, tachypnoea, high BP, visual hallucinations, tremor, confusion, fits.

Insomnia and sleep disorders

Data gathering

Time course	Acute vs. chronic Every day vs. occasionally Difficulty falling asleep vs. interrupted sleep vs. early morning waking Sleeping routine – when go to bed/wakeup? Sleep during day?
Ideas	*"Do you have any idea why you have difficulty sleeping?"* • Stressor, e.g. family, at work, finances, stressful event • Symptom, e.g. cough, pain, apnoea, nocturia • Stimulants, e.g. caffeine Previous treatments tried
Social history	Home, work, relationships, finances Smoking, alcohol, recreational drugs, caffeine
Red flags	Depression and anxiety screen Drug abuse, alcoholism Hypothyroidism Hyperthyroidism
Examination	

Interpersonal skills

ICE	Open questions at the beginning followed by listening will often give you the context for insomnia without you having to ask all the specifics Effect on life, e.g. problems during the day concentrating, driving Important to establish early on what patient wants from doctor and use this to guide management

Management

Investigations	Often none required, TFTs Investigations directed by cause

Management	Treat cause
	
	Conservative
	    Sleep hygiene (see **Tired all the time**)
	    Avoid caffeine and alcohol
	    Symptom diary can be helpful
	Medical
	    Sedative medications (e.g. zopiclone, temazepam)
	    • usually only prescribe for 1 week at a time
	    • explain risks:
	      • long term: addiction, tolerance, cognitive impairment, ataxia
	      • short term: hangover effects, daytime drowsiness and impaired judgement

Safety net	Review as appropriate

Note: whilst alcohol is a sedative, it also causes disrupted sleep patterns.

Eating disorders

Based on NICE guidelines (2004)

Data gathering

Screening	*"Do you think you have an eating problem?"*
	 "Do you worry excessively about your weight?"
	 Symptoms
	     Bingeing, purging, laxatives
	     Restriction diet, exercise
	     Body image, fear fatness
	     Periods, thyroid, GIT
	 Past medical history
	     Depression, anxiety, other psychiatric history

Social history	Work, home, relationships
Red flags	BMI < 60% of normal Poor social support, co-morbidities (psychiatric/ physical), pregnancy
Examination	Weight, BMI, Pulse, BP Mental state

Interpersonal skills

ICE	Importance of gaining rapport and patient's trust Empathy, non-judgemental attitude Issues of confidentiality if patient is a child

Management

Investigations	U&Es, DEXA

Management	Support patient, reassure that assistance is available
	 Conservative
	     Food diary
	     Self help programme
	     Family therapies for children/adolescents
	     Support groups
	 Psychological
	     CBT – refer early
	 Medical
	     SSRI – e.g. fluoxetine 60 mg daily (higher dose than for depression)

Safety net	Monitor extensively if type I diabetes or pregnant
	Admit if weight < 60% of normal

"*Laxative abuse does not greatly reduce calorie absorption*".

After vomiting:

- avoid brushing
- rinse with non-acid mouthwash

Opiate addiction

Data gathering

History	Establish patient's agenda, e.g.: • wanting opiates to prevent withdrawal • wanting help for stabilisation / detoxification • other, e.g. finances, housing Ever injected drugs? Shared needles? Hepatitis B? *Collateral history* From psychiatrist, drug treatment centre, another GP
Social history	Housing, finances Smoking, alcohol, recreational drugs
Red flags	Pregnancy, child protection issues
Examination	Pulse, BP Injection sites, infection / sepsis, opiate withdrawal

Interpersonal skills

ICE	Reassure patient either you and/or a specialist centre will help support him Effectively deal with aggression or demanding patient without provoking patient

Management

Investigations	Urine – drugs screen Bloods – Hep B and C, HIV

Management	Smoking is safer than injection
	Conservative
	    Support groups
	    Needle exchange programmes, don't share needles, safe needle disposal
	    Hepatitis B immunisation
	Medical
	    Methadone or buprenophine stabilisation / detoxification
	    As a general rule do not prescribe opiates on first encounter
	    Treat withdrawal symptoms as needed, e.g. propranolol, loperamide
	Social
	    Benefits, accommodation, occupation, sick notes

| *Safety net* | Refer if complex case or depending on local service agreements |

Opiate withdrawal

Symptoms: abdominal pain, agitation, diarrhoea, dilated pupils, rhinorhoea, sweating, vomiting.

Remember patients cannot die from withdrawal symptoms (although they may feel they will) but they can die from methadone/opiate overdose.

Cannabis abuse

Data gathering

History	How often? Method (smoked, eaten)? Setting? Why started? Any problems encountered? *Screen for harmful effects* See below *Past medical history* Cardiovascular disease Psychiatric history
Social history	Occupation, use of heavy machinery, driving Smoking, alcohol, other recreational drugs, intravenous drug use
Red flags	Dependence, schizophrenia
Examination	Weight, BP, pulse

Interpersonal skills

ICE	Effect on life, relationships, occupation Screen for anxiety and depression Some heavy users may have financial difficulties
To patient	Explain potential harmful effects of use (see below)

Management

Investigations	Consider urine toxicology screen
Management	Advise on stopping Advise on harmful effects, written information Advise regarding law: • illegal • Home Secretary currently recommends reclassification from Class C to Class B drug
Safety net	Review social and financial support

Harmful effects of cannabis

- Cognition: memory loss, irritability.
- Respiratory: cough, wheeze, recurrent respiratory infection.
- Schizophrenia: delusions, hallucinations, delusions of thought control.
- Problems with fertility.
- Dependence, tolerance.

Post-traumatic stress disorder

Based on NICE guidelines (2005)

Data gathering

History	PTSD occurs after exceptionally threatening event, e.g. rape, assault, torture, road traffic accident (i.e. not after divorce, failing exams or loss of job)
	Three main features:
	    1. flashbacks, nightmares – often vivid
	    2. avoidance behaviour – avoid similar situations
	    3. emotional numbing or hyper-arousal
	Also irritability, anger

Social history	Occupation (higher incidence in those working for the military, police, and emergency services) Alcohol, recreational drugs
Red flags	Risk of suicide and deliberate self harm Risk of harming others
Examination	Mental state

Interpersonal skills

ICE	Depression screen, may experience grief, effect on life Consider screening for PTSD in those at high risk

Management

Investigations	

Management	If <4 weeks since event, manage with watchful waiting (unless very severe symptoms)
	Conservative
	    Encourage family involvement if possible
	    Support groups
	    Treat any drug abuse before treating PTSD
	Psychological
	    Trauma-focused CBT
	    Eye movement desensitisation and reprocessing
	Medical
	    Drug treatment not first line, generally to be initiated by specialist
	    e.g. paroxetine, mirtazepine
	    Short-term sedatives may be required for sleep disturbance

Safety net	Regular review for patient support
	Generally needs referral for specialist assessment and treatment
	Beware red flags

Appendix 1 – Influenza and pneumococcal vaccination, AAA screening

Influenza vaccine

Yearly to:
* >65s
* chronic disease: respiratory (including asthma), CHD, chronic renal failure, diabetes
* immunosuppressed: e.g. asplenia
* nursing home residents and carers
* healthcare professionals

Pneumococcal vaccine

Routine childhood vaccine.
Once to adult, booster to high risk (e.g. nephrotic syndrome, asplenia).

AAA screening

Not on NHS, one abdominal ultrasound scan >65 years saves lives (63% mortality reduction).

Appendix 2 – History taking

Cardiovascular history

- Chest pain
- SOB – exertion, orthopnoea, PND
- Palpitations
- Syncope, pre-syncope
- Ankle oedema

Cardiovascular risk factors:
- modifiable: smoking, hypertension, raised cholesterol
- partially-modifiable: family history or past medical history of CVD, CKD, DM, PVD
- non-modifiable: male, increasing age, South Asian origin

Ask about respiratory symptoms.

Respiratory history

- Cough
- Shortness of breath
- Wheeze
- Sputum / haemoptysis
- Chest pain

Gastro-intestinal history

- Abdominal pain
- Nausea, vomiting, diarrhoea
- Weight loss, appetite, diet
- Bowel habit, bleeding
- Consider ectopic in all female patients with abdominal pains

Ask about GU symptoms

Genito-urinary history

Irritative: dysuria, urgency, frequency, incontinence (stress vs. urge)
Obstructive: hesitancy, dribbling/poor stream, nocturia
Haematuria
Vaginal discharge (women)

Obstetric and gynacology history (women)
Sexual history
Ask about GI symptoms

Pain history

Site
Onset
Character
Radiation
Alleviating factors
Time course
Exacerbating factors
Signs and symptoms associated

"Have you ever had this before?"
"Have you tried anything to help the pain? (any medication?)"
ICE

Abdominal pain history

- Relationship to food
- Could patient be pregnant – LMP, unprotected sexual intercourse, etc.
- GI symptoms
- GU symptoms

+/– examining hernial orifices, external genitalia, PR, bimanual
+/– urine dip/MSU

Diagnoses – DKA, glaucoma, migraine

Gynaecology history

Most important are:
- pregnancy (including ectopic)
- STI risk
- periods – LMP, how many days between periods (most and fewest days), how many days bleeding
- contraception
- last smear

Ask yourself: could patient be pregnant? e.g. feeling faint, vomiting, weight gain.

Obstetric history

- Pregnancies
- Miscarriage
- Termination of pregnancy
- Caesarean sections
- Consider post-natal depression for obstetric cases

Sexual history

- Ascertain risk of pregnancy or STI
- Sexually active? With who? Regular partner?
- Use condom? Contraception?
- Any accidents? Missed pill?
- Are you worried about STI?
- Pain? Discharge?
- Does partner have any symptoms?
- LMP?